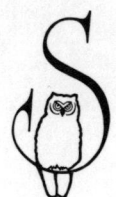

also by Adeline Garner Shell
  Supermarket Counter Power
  American Cookery

also by Kay Reynolds
  Practical Book of Food Shopping
    (with Helen Stone Hovey)

Feel Better After 50 Food Book

Adeline Garner Shell
Kay Reynolds

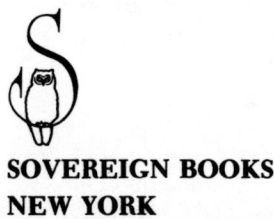

SOVEREIGN BOOKS
NEW YORK

COPYRIGHT © 1978 BY ADELINE GARNER SHELL
ALL RIGHTS RESERVED
INCLUDING THE RIGHT OF REPRODUCTION
IN WHOLE OR IN PART IN ANY FORM
PUBLISHED BY SOVEREIGN BOOKS
A SIMON & SCHUSTER DIVISION OF
GULF & WESTERN CORPORATION
SIMON & SCHUSTER BUILDING
1230 AVENUE OF THE AMERICAS
NEW YORK, NEW YORK 10020
DESIGNED BY DAVID NETTLES
MANUFACTURED IN THE UNITED STATES OF AMERICA
10 9 8 7 6 5 4 3 2 1

LIBRARY OF CONGRESS CATALOGING IN PUBLICATION DATA

Shell, Adeline Garner.
  Feel better after 50 food book.

  Bibliography: p.
  Includes index.
  1. Middle age—Nutrition. 2. Aged—Nutrition.
I. Reynolds, Kay, 1911-   joint author. II. Title.
III. Series.
TX361.M47S53   613.2   78-6748

ISBN 0-671-18370-2
ISBN 0-671-18343-5 paper

Contents

1. How It All Started: The Feel Better Group 3
2. Some Foods You Can't Afford to Miss 8
3. Eat a Real Meal 13
4. What's for Lunch? 20
5. Breakfast: Morning, Noon, or Night 26
6. Think in Threes 31
7. The Handy Food Finder 39
8. A Simple Eating Guide 79
9. Fourteen Days of Feel-Better Food: Passkeys to Livelier Living 86
10. Never Have to Diet Again 102
11. Constipation and Other Problems 124
12. The Feel-Better Kitchen: How to Plan for It 130
13. The Feel-Better Kitchen: How to Buy for It 149
14. The Feel-Better Shopper 170
15. The Feel-Better Cookbook 190

Recommended Reading 207

Index 211

*Feel Better
After 50
Food Book*

1
How It All Started: The Feel Better Group

RECENTLY, an experimental workshop for older people was held in a Queens, New York, multiservice center. It was called the Feel-Better Group. And that was its sole purpose ... to help older people to feel better, mainly through eating better. Adeline Garner Shell, the group's leader, set out to show that eating in the best way to suit your time of life is bound to make a great difference in the way you feel.

Some members of the Feel-Better Group who went home and tried Mrs. Shell's ideas showed a remarkable change. They seemed to find new life. Their skin and hair looked different. They no longer slumped in their chairs. Their spirits, which had been very low, leaped high. "I haven't laughed like this in twenty years!" exclaimed the oldest member of the group, a tiny, intelligent eighty-year-old.

People of many different backgrounds were in the group: Poles, Russians, Scots, Hispanics, Irish, Blacks from the Caribbean islands and the South, Germans, Italians, Jews, and English. Here's how they talked:

"I feel lousy!"
"I always have a headache."
"No ambition."

"Too weak to get out of bed in the morning."
"No pep."
"I am always in some kind of pain."
"I hate being so fat but I don't know how to change."
"I am so constipated!" "Me, too!"—from all but one member.
"I have awful indigestion."
"I feel bored."
"I'm tired all the time so I never go anywhere."
"I'm so thin, I feel nervous and jumpy, but I can't seem to put on a pound."

As a group, these people certainly needed to feel better.

"It just doesn't have to be this way," Mrs. Shell responded, "but it will take us some time to change it. Hang on, because we are all going to feel better if we really want to."

Feel-Bad Diets

When asked what they were eating, very few reported a good diet that would help the body to work well.

"I have a hot meal in the middle of the day, and then I only need peanut butter and crackers at night."
"I don't feel like cooking just for myself so when I get hungry, I have doughnuts and coffee, and that fills me up."
"I know what foods I need, but I can't afford them on my income now that I'm older."
"What can you buy that's in portions for one person? If you live alone, you just can't eat right."
"I get up too late to eat breakfast. It's already time for lunch."
"I really like fresh vegetables but everything comes in such large packages, I never buy them anymore."

It was evident that for these people to feel better by eating better, many problems would have to be solved. It was relatively easy to show through interesting demonstrations with real food just what kind of food was needed to enable the after-fifty eater to feel better. But how was a person living alone to buy, prepare, and store food in ways to permit a good variety, including fresh foods? How was waste to be avoided? How could the food nutrients be preserved for second- or third-time servings? In lively demonstration sessions, Mrs. Shell showed the skills and know-how needed to take good care of yourself.

Feeling Better about Food Money

For those who felt they couldn't afford good food, and for those who wanted to save money on food so they could spend it on other things to make life more pleasant, Mrs. Shell demonstrated many ways of making choices among foods to save a lot of money. Her special way of buying and preparing meat was shown. It saves $72.00 a year in itself.

"What could you do with $72 extra right now?" Mrs. Shell asked the group.

"I'd buy the clothes I need."
"I'd go on a vacation."
"Just to have an extra dollar on you is good!"
"I'd pay my doctor bills."
"I'd save $60 and spend the rest on myself!"
"I'd buy a coat which I don't need but it would give me pleasure."
"I'd take a trip to Florida in the cold weather."

Other money-saving sessions that the group enjoyed were Mrs. Shell's ways to get the most for the money at the supermarket.

Change Takes Time

Not everybody in the group did everything at once. Change takes time, especially when you're older. Revolutions are made by the young. The older go slower. Some members overcame their constipation. Naturally they felt better than they had for years. They left till later the changes that would bring about large savings in their food bills by better ways of planning, shopping for, storing, and preparing food. Some people started drinking milk, and found that this alone made a great difference in their energy and well-being. Some found out how to reduce sensibly, and were thrilled to gradually shed their fat. They, too, saved other aspects of feeling better about food for later.

"Out of all these ideas, take the ones that suit you best," Mrs. Shell advised, "and build on them."

A Real Life Approach

The Feel-Better Group were encouraged to ask questions whenever they felt like it. They did. Some of their questions suggested the most valuable chapters in this book. It's a book based on real experience, not theory.

As the group moved into its later sessions, and a really practical knowledge of nutrition for the older years was gained, one member, looking back on a life of poor eating and fearing damage to her body, inquired "Is it too late for us?"

"No, it's not too late," Mrs. Shell replied. "We're going to live a long time, perhaps another twenty years for some of us; for others, even longer. No matter how long we live, we want to feel the best we know how, and to be as healthy as possible. Good eating helps that. When you feel better, you can feel better for others, too, that is, you can *do* for others . . . and that always makes a person feel better!"

Cooking for One

The cooking-for-one sessions were magnets for the members of the center. Several people in the group, after tasting Mrs. Shell's homemade bread, wanted to make their own, for better eating and for the pleasure of it. But some were arthritic and didn't feel they had enough strength in their arms to bear down on the bread dough to knead it. Mrs. Shell introduced them to a simple but delicious casserole bread that required no kneading at all, and they've been baking the No-Knead Breads happily ever since.

Those attending these sessions got up when they saw what was going on, and brought in others by the hand so they could share and learn, too. These were happy times and they are all reflected in this book in dozens of menus, recipes, ideas for feeling better, the best foods, and how they work in the body.

Food Is No Cure-All

Food can make you feel better, Mrs. Shell assured the group, but it will not change some things that we must learn to live with in our later years. As we grow older, many changes take place in our bodies. Our eyesight isn't as good. Our body doesn't burn food as well as it did because the metabolism slows down. We have to take into consideration that our well-being is affected by past illnesses, accidents, infections, and all the other experiences that a body goes through in a lifetime. When you add a poor diet to these conditions, it is easy to understand why many older people do *not* feel better.

The older years are often a time of turmoil, of trying to learn to live with changes. They may be very serious, such as the death of a mate. Many of these things must be accepted. But the one thing you, and you alone, *can* control is the way that you eat. You can make a change for the better here that will make a big difference. Better food gives you the energy to walk, to move, to breathe, to keep the heart beating, to keep the muscles working in the most efficient way for you.

Older people must reduce their calorie intake by 150 to 200 calories a day compared with the number consumed when they were between 35 and 50 years old. Because the metabolism changes and older people are usually less active, the same amount of food cannot be handled. That's why it is important that each and every food eaten give the maximum nutrition. There's no room for foods with high calories but low food value. Every bite must count. For people who have never been sure how to eat right, now is the time to learn the feel-better way. Let's begin.

2
Some Foods You Can't Afford to Miss

People in the feel-better group soon found that they had been missing out on a lot of important foods in their meals. Putting these foods back in the diet quickly helped them to feel better. What foods are older people leaving out?

They're Leaving Out the "Leafies"

Green leafy vegetables like spinach and collards, as well as broccoli, are needed daily, or at least every other day, for people to feel their best.

Why? They have vitamin A. This helps to keep the skin wet inside the body. When this skin dries out, as it can without enough vitamin A foods, people are more likely to get infections from germs. The wet skin inside the body forms a shield that keeps germs from invading.

A half-cup of most cooked green leafy vegetables gives people more than enough vitamin A for the day. Equally good vitamin A foods are dark orange vegetables, such as carrots and sweet potatoes which may be used in place of the "green leafies." These foods also have fiber, or roughage, which is important for good elimination.

They're Leaving Out Bread and Cereals

Because of silly reducing diets, people think that bread is fattening, and we have found that many people are omitting it from their daily meals. Here are the facts. A slice of enriched white bread has an average of only 75 calories, and a slice of whole wheat bread only 65 calories.

What happens when people leave bread out of their meals? They are missing an inexpensive source of thiamine, riboflavin, niacin, and iron. These nutrients are absolutely essential to good health.

The word *nutrients* is just a shorthand term that scientists use for referring to the good things in food that are nourishing and help to keep people healthy. You've heard a lot about vitamins. Vitamin A. Vitamin C. And others. They are nutrients. So is protein. So is iron. A food may be high or low in nutrients. It's easier to say it that way than to give a long list of what each nutrient is every time a food is mentioned.

Breakfast cereals, both hot and cold, are also left out of the diet by older people because they think they are high in calories. But here's the truth. A 1-ounce serving of ready-to-eat cereal has 110 calories, without milk and sugar. A cup of cooked oatmeal, 130 calories. A cup of cooked, enriched regular farina has only 105 calories. Serving it with a half-cup of whole milk adds only 75 calories; with skim milk, only 45 calories. The sugar can be skipped, but even if it is used, there are only 15 calories in a level teaspoon. To sum up, a cup of cooked farina served with a half-cup of skim milk and one level teaspoon of sugar gives you only 165 calories.

Few people realize that cereals are one of the lowest calorie main dishes to serve at breakfast. By comparison, a plain Danish (called sweet roll in some localities) has 275 calories and doesn't supply the good things that are in cereals.

When people eat bread and cereals that are made from whole grains such as whole wheat rather than enriched white flour, they get special benefits. For instance, 100 grams of whole wheat flour has 2.3 grams of fiber whereas enriched all-purpose white flour has only 0.3 grams. That is more than seven times more fiber in whole wheat flour than in white flour. No doubt you've been reading that fiber, or roughage, is believed to be more and more important to the smooth working of the body. In addition, in whole grain foods, you get some nutrients that are lost during the processing of white flour, and which are not put back in white flour even when it is enriched.

They're Leaving Out Milk

Milk is not just kid stuff, as many people believe.

In a modern-day diet, unless milk and foods made from it, such as cheese, are included, it is almost impossible to get the calcium needed for healthy bones and teeth, the proper clotting of the blood, the water balance in the body, and the proper muscle contractions and nerve responses, so important to feeling well. If all these things don't work right, how can a person possibly feel good?

Fortified vitamin D milk, and foods made from this milk, are not only rich in calcium but are also inexpensive sources of protein and riboflavin. Did you know that just two glasses of milk provide 45 percent of the protein, 55 percent of the riboflavin, and 75 percent of the calcium for one day of the USRDA (United States Recommended Daily Allowances). The USRDA's are the amounts of protein, vitamins, and minerals established by the Food and Drug Administration as standards for nutrition labeling. These allowances are based on the Recommended Daily Dietary Allowances set by the Food and Nutrition Board of the National Research Council.

Milk is absolutely essential to a feel-better diet for a normally healthy person. For that small group which cannot tolerate milk, it is best to turn to a physician for advice on alternate sources of calcium.

They're Leaving Out Raw Fruits and Vegetables

Fruits and vegetables are excellent fiber foods, especially when eaten raw. They are a fine balance to the large amount of refined, or overprocessed, foods eaten by most people today.

Besides scrubbing out the insides, raw fruits and vegetables help to free the teeth of sticky foods such as gravy, syrups, and other heavily sugared foods. To feel better, it is best to eat some raw foods at least twice a day. This also supplies vitamins and minerals, texture, new taste sensations, and stimulates the appetite.

Most fruits are best eaten raw. Many vegetables are too. Have you ever tried sliced raw asparagus, raw peas, broccoli cut in very small pieces, shredded red or regular cabbage, carrots, radishes, spinach leaves, thinly sliced zucchini? For those who feel this is too much raw food, try combining some of the raw vegetables with cooked vegetables in a salad. For example, add cooked carrots and peas to a salad made with mixed greens. Those who mix and match raw and cooked vegetables will have dozens of new salads at their table.

Most important, a mixture of the right vegetables will provide daily meals with significant amounts of vitamin A, vitamin C, thiamine, riboflavin, iron, and in some instances, calcium. For example, one medium stalk of broccoli provides 45 calories, 90 percent of the vitamin A needed daily, over 100 percent of the vitamin C, 13 percent of the thiamine, 22 percent of the riboflavin, 17 percent of the niacin, 19 percent of the calcium, and 13 percent of the iron. Broccoli is a blockbuster vegetable for feel-better diets.

Some people may have been told at one time that they should not eat raw foods because they have diverticulitis or other intestinal disturbances. It would be advisable to check again with a doctor since recent medical research has influenced many physicians into changing their recommendations about the use of raw vegetables and fruits in such cases. In fact, some researchers feel it may be helpful rather than harmful to eat raw fruits and vegetables under these conditions. Be sure to check with the doctor, however, before making any change.

They're Leaving Out Foods Rich in Vitamin C

To feel better, people need vitamin C foods such as grapefruit and cabbage each and every day. Vitamin C is not stored by the body as many other nutrients are.

Important signs of vitamin C shortage in adults are listlessness, lack of endurance, small hemorrhages under the skin, gums which bleed easily, and fleeting pains in the legs and joints. These pains are often mistaken for rheumatism.

To make meal planning easier and food shopping more economical, it is important to know that two good food sources of vitamin C can be combined to take the place of one high vitamin C food. For example, if a potato, boiled in the skin, or baked, and a serving of coleslaw, are eaten in one day, the daily vitamin C needs will be more than met.

Many more good foods are left out of average diets by older people, too many to cover here. We will deal with all of them in turn so that you won't be missing a thing that is good for you.

In chapter 7, "The Handy Food Finder" tells in detail all about the good things in food, which foods have them, and what they do for you. It shows which foods have the most vitamin C, vitamin A, protein, and all the other nutrients needed daily. This is a good guide to help get together the right kind of foods for each day. There is a shorter guide in chapter 8. Now for some other important things to know about feel-better eating.

3
Eat a Real Meal

IN THIS AGE OF FAST FOODS and frozen dishes, many people have forgotten what a real meal is.

Some of the most popular places to eat—the fast-food hamburger chains—never serve a real meal. It's only part of a meal. A hamburger on a bun, for instance. All the other parts of a real meal, such as vegetables, fruits, and milk are missing. This doesn't give you the full nourishment that you need. A meal like this is like a flower with half the petals pulled off. It's a mutilated meal. It's not complete.

It's bad enough that people don't eat a real meal when they eat out. But it's even worse that so many persons have copied fast food meals at home. As a result, they hardly ever have a real meal—even at dinner—and are seriously undernourished. That's where the "no pep," "always tired" feelings often come from. Ads, TV commercials, billboards, all show you in glorious color a meal that isn't a real meal. No wonder people are influenced to eat against their best interests.

One reason why it's important for people to eat at home as often as they can is to get real meals made with all the foods needed, in the right combinations. When people take this first step, they soon begin to feel better.

Here are three favorite American meals:

Hamburger on a Bun
French Fries
Cola Drink

Slice of Pizza
Cola Drink

Cold Cuts
Potato Salad
Pickles
Rolls
Cola Drink
(the "deli" meal)

These may be favorite meals but will they help you to feel better?

How to Make a Dinner with Hamburger

A ground-beef patty is a fine food for dinner, but don't eat it as a hamburger in a big, soft white roll. That's too much bread for an older person to eat at one meal. It fills you up so fast you don't have room for the other good foods needed in a real meal. Forget the hamburger roll and eat instead a slice of bread with dinner. Whole wheat bread is preferable, but it's not a must. Now there's room for the other good foods in a hamburger dinner. Put them all together in a simple feel-better meal like this:

Hamburger Patty
Boiled Potato
Broccoli
Bread
Fruit Cup
Cup of Milk

Besides changing from a roll to bread, other good-for-you foods are added: vegetables, fruit, milk.

A real meal like this gives you half the day's needs of protein, calcium, and some vitamins at one meal. If it strikes you as being too much food to eat at one time, save the fruit cup and milk for a snack later on.

One of the leading fast-food chains features a quarter-pound hamburger for 85 cents. It seems cheap, but think of it this way: you can buy enough beef for three quarter-pound hamburgers to make at home for about the price of a single hamburger on a roll at this chain. When you plan your food this way, you start to feel better about your food money. You spend a lot less and you eat a lot better.

None of this is to knock the hamburger as a good food. Often when you have to lunch out, a hamburger is the best choice for your money. But don't depend upon it for dinner. Come on home for that.

Vote No for Hamburger and French Fries

As for the favorite combination of hamburger and french fries, that's a no-no for older people who want to feel better.

Potatoes are a wonderful food, but they're best for older people when eaten plain, either boiled or baked in the skin. Add a bit of butter or margarine, if you like. Complete the meal with vegetable, fruit, and milk along with the meat.

French fries could be said to be maimed potatoes. They burden the body with unneeded fat, and are often more difficult for an older person to digest than a plain potato. When an equal amount of potato cooked in the skin is compared with the same amount of french fried potatoes, there are *three times* as many calories in the french fries! It's because of the fat. Older people can't afford these extra calories since they leave no room for other important foods that provide what is needed for good health. So remember, eat potatoes in the nude (the potatoes, not you!)—they're better for you.

Cola Is Not a Feel-Better Beverage

You'll notice that in our real-meal hamburger menu, no cola drink was included despite the fact that a favorite

American meal is hamburger, french fries and a cola drink. Why did we leave it out? Because when people drink cola, they're really wasting calories. Cola drink counts for absolutely nothing but energy value. The 90 calories in a cup of regular cola drink come from sugar and/or other sweeteners. A cup of skim milk has 90 calories. However, these calories give 22 percent of the protein needed for the day, 28 percent of the riboflavin, and 37 percent of the calcium, plus small amounts of other nutrients. It's important to choose a drink that adds up to feeling better.

Can You Make a Real Meal with Store-Bought Pizza?

Yes. But only a lunch, not a dinner. And not a very good lunch at that, unless you add other foods to the meal. As our nutrition-wise Spanish friend tells her children, *"Pizza no es una comida!"* (Pizza is not a meal.)

Pizza doesn't have enough good things in it to be a wise choice for a main dish. For instance, a slice of pizza has only 10 percent of the protein needed for a day. Protein, as you probably know, is essential to build, maintain, and repair the body's muscles, tissues, and cells. In contrast to pizza, just a 1-ounce slice of American cheese has 15 percent of the protein needed for a day, and one tiny clam fritter has as much protein as a whole slice of pizza!

People should treat pizza as a snack food. But if they choose to have it for lunch, here is a menu that helps to make it a real meal:

> Slice of Pizza
> Mixed Green Salad
> Stewed Fruit
> Cup of Milk

Pizza is a good example of how carefully people have to look into the foods they buy to decide which ones are worth eating after fifty.

Pizza is likely to have only a sprinkling of cheese on top and that isn't enough to make a good main dish. If you buy your pizza at a pizzeria, watch them when they're making one up. They may be generous with the cheese and if so your pizza will be more nourishing. If not, keep trying pizzerias—you may find one that really gives you a good deal with the cheese.

As for buying frozen pizza at the supermarket, which so many do, check labels very carefully to see what you are eating. It may not be a feel-better choice. Reading labels is one of the best ways of making sure to get the best food for a feel-better diet.

Here's a label from a pizza that is sold in supermarkets all over the United States. Check it out. Notice how many of the things used to make this pizza are imitation foods or chemicals substituting for food:

Frozen Peperoni* Pizza Ingredients (13 ounces)

Crust. Wheat flour, water, peanut oil, sugar, yeast, nonfat dry milk, calcium propionate, corn meal.

Sauce. Tomatoes, water, tomato sauce mix (dehydrated tomato flakes, modified starch, potato flour, salt, monosodium glutamate, sugar, beet powder, citric acid, artificial certified color), corn oil, salt, spices, vegetable gums (guar gum, gum tragacanth), garlic.

Blended Topping. Imitation mozzarella cheese (water, saturated soya oil, potassium caseinate, sodium caseinate, salt, lactic acid, lipolyzed butter oil, potassium sorbate added as a preservative, artificial certified color), low moisture part-skim mozzarella cheese.

Peperoni. Pork, beef, salt, spices, sugar, paprika, sodium ascorbate, sodium nitrate, garlic powder, sodium nitrite.

---

* Peperoni is a hard, dry Italian sausage, often used in traditional pizza.

People who read this label can see for themselves that there are better choices for a feel-better meal. As members of the Feel-Better Group learned how to read labels, they were able to buy better foods and often reported their finds with pleased excitement.

To return to pizza. If you make your own pizza at home, it's quite another story! And it's easy to do. You don't have to make a pizza dough as they do in the store. With the special recipes given on pages 198-200, you can make a whole pizza or individual portions, and have a protein-rich main dish that fits the feel-better plan. Homemade pizza tastes just great with its fresh, simple ingredients, and plenty of them.

Can You Make a Real Meal with Cold Cuts?

A favorite meal with some of the Feel-Better Group people was cold cuts like bologna and old-fashioned loaf, potato salad, pickle, roll and cola drink. What's missing here? There are no green or yellow vegetables, no salad for vitamins and minerals, and no milk to drink. It's not a real meal.

Besides, as the feel-better people discovered, cold cuts are not the best meat choice when the protein value of cold cuts is compared to such foods as American pasteurized cheese, an equal amount of fresh beef, cottage cheese, macaroni and cheese, homemade chili con carne, or scrambled eggs. Two ounces of bologna (three thin slices) provide 16 percent protein in comparison to 33 percent in a 2-ounce serving of cooked hamburger. That's twice as much protein in the beef as in the bologna!

You can make a better meal, a real meal, with any of the above-mentioned foods than with cold cuts. Ham, roast beef, turkey are delicatessen cold cuts with good food value but they are very expensive. For the same money, people can get a lot more food of equally good quality.

Most cold cuts have a salt content too high for older people. Their fat content is also high, and they have sweeteners such as corn syrup and dextrose which give unneeded calories, and additives that are currently under investigation.

When a person feels like having a cold dinner—perhaps on a very hot day—what would make a real meal instead of cold cuts? If a delicious homemade meat loaf is on hand, serve a slice or two of that for a nourishing cold main dish and build a real meal around it for dinner. Meat loaf is so easy to make. Freeze it in individual portions to keep in the freezer or freezing compartment of the refrigerator. It will be ready to defrost and serve any time a cold meal is wanted. There's a fabulous recipe for meat loaf on page 192.

Here's a cold meal that combines feel-better foods:

    Homemade Meat Loaf
    Potato Salad
    Mixed Green Salad with Grated Carrot and Tomato
    Bread
    Apple
    Cup of Milk   Tea

Here's another good cold meal:

    Platter of Cheese Slices
    Macaroni Salad
    Sliced Tomato
    Carrot Sticks
    Whole Wheat Bread
    Pear or Other Fruit
    Tea

In this menu, the cheese, a dairy product made from milk, takes the place of milk to drink. This meal can be changed easily by using either tuna or chicken salad in place of the cheese slices. If these changes are made, add a cup of milk to the meal.

There's a great deal more to tell. So much more to enjoy. So many ways of feeling better. You'll find delicious dinners in chapter 9, "Fourteen Days of Feel-Better Food," all worked out to give the good things needed at the main meal. In chapter 15, there are great recipes to match the meals, made with the best of foods for the least money. But now let's have a look at lunch.

4
What's for Lunch?

HERE ARE SOME LUNCHES that we have found popular with older people. Cream cheese sandwich. Tuna sandwich. Peanut butter sandwich. Canned spaghetti. Pea soup. Chicken noodle soup. Hot dog. And then there is the "nothing" lunch—nothing at all!

Most of these foods are good foods, but they can't stand all by themselves to make a good lunch. A few simple additions are needed to make them feel-better lunches.

A sandwich is a very good luncheon dish. But the feel-better people learned to look in the middle to make sure it was a feel-better filling. Cream cheese doesn't quite fill the bill. The facts are that cream cheese has about 8 percent protein, 51 percent water, and about 37 percent fat. Compare this with the same amount of Cheddar cheese, or rat cheese, as some people call it. It has about 25 percent protein, 37 percent water, 32 percent fat, and more than ten times as much calcium as cream cheese. Remember, the body must have protein and calcium every day. Cream cheese for lunch isn't the best way to get them.

As for the peanut butter and tuna sandwiches, they are good food. But they need a little company to make them into the feel-better lunch. Here's one way to do it:

What's for Lunch? • 21

> Peanut Butter-Raisin Sandwich
> Fruit Cup of Banana, Orange, Peach,
>   or Other Fruit in Season
> Cup of Milk

That's a really nourishing noontime meal. Now what has been added? A few raisins are stirred into the peanut butter to add iron, a mineral often missing in older people's diets. Fresh fruits have been added for vitamins and bulk. And don't forget the milk. In this lunch, it is particularly important because the protein in peanut butter is incomplete, and it has to be improved by a complete protein food in order for the body to use it well. Milk, a complete protein food, does that job in this menu.

As for the tuna sandwich, tuna is a complete protein food so the menu is a little different. The milk is not needed to improve the protein quality of the tuna.

> Tomato Juice
> Tuna Sandwich
> Pear or Any Fresh Fruit in Season
> Coffee or Tea

Of course, milk should be part of other meals during the day.

Soup, Soup, Beautiful Soup?

Pea soup, another luncheon favorite, is good but, like the peanut butter, it doesn't have complete protein so it needs a companion food. Just add a quarter-cup of diced cooked beef or pork to the soup, and that does it. To round out the meal, have a carrot and raisin salad, a thin slice of bread, an orange or your favorite fruit, and a cup of milk.

Soups like canned chicken noodle soup or chicken rice soup have very little protein. They don't make good main dishes for lunch unless you add to them some of your own cooked chicken and vegetables. In addition, eat a slice of bread, fresh fruit, and drink a glass of milk.

How about canned spaghetti for lunch? It sure is a big temptation to just open a can and heat the food. But what is it doing for you? Canned spaghetti doesn't give enough protein for the noonday meal. Enrich it yourself. Add a small amount of diced cheese on top, or stir in a small amount of cooked beef, pork, or chicken. Round out this meal with a green salad, fruit, and milk.

Frankfurters Are an "Iffy" Food

For lunch, frankfurters are an "iffy" food. If you have no other meat to eat, frankfurters are better than none. But we do not feel that frankfurters are the best meat choice for people after fifty. For one thing, most of them are highly salted and a lot of salt is not advisable in the diets of older people. Frankfurters are very spicy and by law they may contain up to 30 percent fat and 10 percent water. Hamburgers, too, may contain up to 30 percent fat, but there's a difference in the eating. The hamburger fat cooks out and is discarded. The fat in frankfurters stays within the skin casing for the most part, and it is eaten.

Besides these undesirable things about frankfurters for older people, there is the fact that nitrites are used in processing frankfurters to kill botulism bacteria and to intensify the red color of the meat. If the nitrite is not used, the frankfurters are gray in appearance. Nitrites are viewed with apprehension by many scientists for their effect on the human system. In some countries, they are forbidden or limited in use.

Frankfurters vary greatly in quality and in the type of meats with which they are made. If you should see a package of frankfurters with meat by-products listed in the ingredients, this is what these meat by-products may be according to the law governing the making of frankfurters: pork stomachs or snouts; beef, veal, lamb or goat tripe; beef, veal, lamb, goat or pork hearts, tongues, fat, lips, esophagus and spleens; and partially defatted pork or beef fatty tissue. It's wise to read labels carefully.

As for cost, comparing franks to ground beef only on a price basis does not give a true picture. The real thing to compare is the amount of protein you get for the money, and this is where we helped our Feel-Better Group to see the difference. There is about twice as much protein in fresh beef as in most frankfurters. Therefore, the beef is usually a less expensive way of getting protein. It's the real food value that counts.

Need any more be said about a hot dog for lunch?

And Now, Ladies and Gentlemen, the Nothing Lunch

This is not a lecture. You've heard it all before. But when you give yourself promises for lunch ("I'll eat something later") instead of food, studies show that it is hardly ever made up during the day. What happens is that people get very hungry and grab for anything in sight—potato chips, a doughnut, cookies, a candy bar, cake, soft drink—which adds unneeded calories without the other good things that are an important part of feeling better.

Not only do people eat inferior foods, but they're so hungry they usually eat more than if they had had a good, well-planned meal. So the nothing lunch is double jeopardy for older people who want to feel better. Another way to look at it is that if lunch is missed, what should be about one-third of the food needed for the day is lost, and people end up only two-thirds nourished!

If You Work Outside Your Home

This presents a real problem. To eat a lunch that is really good for you, such as those we have given, may be too expensive in a restaurant. The hamburger-and-french-fries lunch prevails in most parts of the United States. When you want something different, it's more work for the restaurant, more service, and you pay for it. What can you do?

The smartest older people are taking their lunch to work. It's a revolution. Companies are providing places for employees to eat because so many bring their own meals. Where that isn't possible, the lounge room for employees or, in good weather, the park, provides a pleasant place to eat.

You can take a well-balanced meal in a lunchbox. And you'll save so much money it will be a sweet bonus. One person saved enough for a vacation by taking lunch to work.

Here are some tote lunches made with feel-better foods:

    Cheese Sandwich
    Whole Tomato
    Fresh Fruit
    Oatmeal Cookie
    Tea or Coffee

Note. If you need more, add homemade vegetable beef soup or canned pea soup carried in a vacuum bottle.

    Cold Sliced Meat Loaf Sandwich
    Carrot and Green Pepper Sticks
    Plums or Other Seasonal Fruit
    Milk

Note. If you need more, add tomato soup.

    Thick Pea Soup
        with Cooked Chopped Beef or Pork Added
    Tomato, Green Pepper, and Celery Salad
    Bread
    Apple or Orange
    Cup of Milk

    Chicken Sandwich
    Coleslaw
    Banana
    Cookies
    Milk

A Hot Main Dish Lunch

    Beef and Vegetable Stew
        (carried in wide-mouth vacuum bottle)
    Slice of Whole Wheat Bread
    Strawberries or Other Fruit in Season
    Milk

Even when older people are on special diets, they can carry their lunch to work. In fact, it is better for them. For instance, those with diabetes, where sugar must be controlled, cannot determine in a restaurant if a salad dressing has sugar added, and if it has, how much. Sugar is often added to gravies, sauces, and other foods where it is not detected easily. Many of the vegetables eaten out are canned and have some sugar added.

In diets where salt is restricted, it is almost impossible to get the proper food outside the home. Because so many restaurants use convenience foods, the salt content of their meals is higher.

For those who are watching their calories, most restaurant meals that fit the pocketbook do not fit the diet. When you carry your own lunches, you eat better, spend less, and provide the right food for your particular situation. A nice little extra is that you can eat the foods you like best, not just what a restaurant offers.

Whether eating lunch at home or at work, never make the mistake of not finding time to sit down and eat a good meal. Eat it in peace and quiet. Refuse to be hurried. You'll feel better!

A good example is that of an older friend who is an office worker in a very busy place. She brings her lunch to the office but, before she eats it, she goes for a short pleasant walk to get away from the tension of the morning's work. She then returns, goes to the company lounge, and has a quiet, peaceful lunch. A bonus is that most of the people in the office eat early and have already left the lounge, so there is not much chance of getting involved in job talk.

If you eat lunch at home, you'll find many good ideas for nourishing and enjoyable noonday meals in chapter 9.

5
Breakfast: Morning, Noon, or Night

AMERICAN BREAKFASTERS may not realize that they have been brainwashed!

On the radio, TV, in magazines, newspapers, the cereal manufacturers keep up a constant hullabaloo. They say that breakfast is fruit, cereal, milk, bread, and spread. That's a good breakfast. Nobody denies it. But people in the Feel-Better Group had come to believe it was the *only* breakfast. Some didn't like it. That turned them off in the morning and they had no breakfast at all.

"I don't like breakfast foods—cereals and stuff like that—so I don't eat breakfast. I just have a cup of coffee—that I like!" That's the way they talked.

We showed them that there are many foods that are great for breakfast, once the TV cereal static is tuned out. Then they began eating breakfast again. Of course, the foods must be good, high in protein, and body-building. You can't just grab a food like a doughnut and call it breakfast.

Eat to Your Taste

Recently while fishing in Westport in the state of Washington, Mrs. Shell met a retired couple who had brought their breakfast with them to eat on the boat. What did they have? A very good breakfast—but no cereal. They had big, fresh salmon sandwiches stuffed with lots of salmon, sliced tomatoes, and green escarole leaves. Then came a banana, and a vacuum bottle of milk. Here was a wonderful breakfast. The people had wisely called up the specially fine foods where they lived. In most cities, a fresh salmon sandwich would be very expensive, but people could enjoy the same type of sandwich using another kind of fish, if they liked it.

While at a campsite in the Grand Canyon, a lady from Texas started her day with homemade chili con carne ("Texas style," she announced proudly), bread, an orange, and special coffee that was half milk. The chili was left over from last night's supper. Here's a good tip: you, too, can make a very good breakfast from dinner leftovers. If you're living alone, this saves a lot of work and planning.

Another good leftover breakfast was enjoyed by a woman from Virginia. She had her favorite Brunswick stew, a specialty of her part of the country, made with chicken, lima beans, corn, tomatoes, and green peppers. It was served with homemade rolls, grapefruit, and milk. What a great breakfast!

In sunny California, one of the favorite after-fifty breakfasts is a big bowl of fresh fruit salad topped with either cottage cheese or yogurt. Served with cinnamon toast and coffee or tea, this is not only a good breakfast but very good-tasting, too.

Here's another point about breakfasts and after-fifty people. Several members of the Feel-Better Group told us that they liked the night hours best for watching late TV shows and doing handwork when it's quiet. They went to bed very late. "When I get up, it isn't time for breakfast. It's time for lunch!" "Then eat lunch," Mrs. Shell advised them. This surprised people because they had been so brainwashed about eating a set kind of breakfast. "But," Mrs. Shell cautioned, "be sure to get that missed meal before you go to bed."

What's a nice late meal to take the place of the missed breakfast? Enjoy an egg prepared a favorite way with a piece of toast and fresh fruit in season. Or how about tomato soup, a cheese sandwich, applesauce, and a glass of milk. Orange juice, a dish of bread pudding with raisins, and a glass of milk make a pleasant "evening breakfast." So does macaroni and cheese with a fresh fruit cup and a glass of milk. Some people who don't enjoy getting up to a cereal breakfast may find it more appealing at night. A bowl of cereal and milk eaten with fruit, or with a glass of juice, is a good nighttime snack. Eat it with a piece of toast to duplicate the missed breakfast in the morning.

Some older people sleep better if they have something hot before going to bed. A bowl of hot cereal like farina or oatmeal, along with a hot milk drink, is a good choice. If a person lives alone, it's cozy and comforting to break up the evening with a nice little meal.

With this plan, people get up, eat lunch, have dinner at the regular time, and then have one of the meals just described. Eat it as late as is comfortable. This way, breakfast is eaten at the other end of the day instead of at a time when a person may not feel like the standard American meal.

If You Eat Breakfast in the Morning

For those who do like to get up and have the advertised breakfast, just be sure to include all the foods—fruit or fruit juice, a cooked or ready-to-eat cereal with milk, a piece of bread such as toast, and milk. This isn't intended to take away the coffee or tea that people like in the morning. Enjoy that, too, along with the milk.

One way to improve a good breakfast is to make coffee half and half: half hot milk and half coffee. In Europe, this is the regular breakfast coffee. They call it *café au lait*—and is it good!

Another good breakfast is fruit, egg, bread, and milk. For variety, part of the milk and the egg can be combined in waffles, pancakes, or French toast. People who don't like eating an egg plain can scramble it, and put it in a sandwich. Use catsup, if you like. That's your pleasure. Don't be hemmed in by what the ads say. Do it to your taste.

There's lots of breakfast variety throughout this great country of ours. Up in Boston town, one of the favorite main dishes is a baked bean sandwich on brown bread made from beans left over from the night before. Often a thin slice of ham is included in this sandwich. Another New England custom for breakfast is to enjoy a big serving of homemade bread pudding, made less sweet than usual. The recipe is on page 204. New Englanders serve their breakfast pudding with fresh fruit or juice, and a warm drink. It's quite handy to have this bread pudding in the refrigerator to serve when a person feels like it. It's very nourishing because it is made with plenty of egg, milk, and bread. And it's so economical.

And now, for those of you who can't always find the time in the morning to have a good breakfast, or have a hard time getting moving, here's a great trick. It's the Feel-Better Breakfast in a Drink (see recipe on next page). When it is drunk along with a slice of toast, it gives everything needed at breakfast. It contains milk (or skim milk), orange juice, banana, vanilla, and a touch of cinnamon or nutmeg. For extra nourishment, add an egg. If eggs are limited in the diet, just add the egg white, or instead, 2 tablespoons of nonfat dry milk. When you use the milk rather than the egg, you increase the amount of calcium in the drink. Some people add a teaspoon of bran or wheat germ. One woman in the Feel-Better Group used a quarter-cup of cottage cheese in place of an egg. Another person suggested using an equal amount of yogurt in place of the milk. Buttermilk fans like the drink better when the milk is replaced with their favorite beverage.

The Feel-Better Breakfast in a Drink gives about 25 percent of the protein, over 75 percent of the vitamin C, 25 percent of the riboflavin, about 15 percent of thiamine, 25 percent of calcium, as well as a small amount of other nutrients needed daily by the after-fifty person.

When an egg is added, the drink then gives slightly over 33 percent of the protein, over 75 percent the vitamin C, about 20 percent the thiamine, 33 percent the riboflavin, and 25 percent the calcium.

You can buzz up this drink in a blender in moments in the morning. If you don't have a blender, you can still make it quickly, using a rotary egg beater. And remember, taken with toast, this is a complete breakfast: all that is needed in the morning to feel better.

For those whose hands are stiff in the morning from arthritis or other ailments, make the drink before going to bed, and put the covered blender container in the refrigerator. Just buzz it up a few moments in the morning and drink it through a wide straw.

Feel-Better Breakfast in a Drink

¾ cup skim or regular whole milk
¼ cup orange juice
1 small or medium, ripe banana, cut into pieces
Vanilla extract to taste
Dash cinnamon or nutmeg

Pour milk and orange juice into blender container. Add banana, vanilla, and spice. Cover and blend until smooth and creamy.

To make with rotary egg beater. Mash banana in a bowl, add orange juice and beat; gradually add the milk, beating after each addition. Add vanilla and spice, and beat.

Variations
1. Add an egg or an egg white
2. Use yogurt or buttermilk instead of regular milk
3. Add 2 or more tablespoons powdered nonfat dry milk
4. Add ¼ cup of cottage cheese
5. Add a teaspoon or more of bran or wheat germ

6
Think in Threes

IT'S TIME TO PAUSE and put things together so far.

Though we have dealt with breakfast, lunch, and dinner separately, the way to feel better is to plan the three meals in a day all at once. No one meal can give all the good things needed in a day. But three meals can, when the foods are planned and put together to add up to just what the body needs in one day to work better. So always think in threes!

It's a good idea to plan dinner first because this meal usually brings the biggest share of the day's food needs. Then to give a good foundation for the coming day, plan breakfast. Let lunch fill in any gaps in the good things needed every day to feel better.

Of course, people new to nutrition—as so many are—won't be able to do this without help right now. But they soon will, using this book. Keep it handy to keep you straight. For now, take these three menus on faith to show how things go together to make you feel better.

A Sample Day of Feel-Better Food

Breakfast
Prunes
Wheat Flakes or Farina with Milk
Whole Wheat Bread with Spread
Coffee Made Half with Milk

Lunch
Vegetable Soup
Cheese Sandwich
Sliced Banana or Peaches
with Milk
Beverage

Dinner
Beef Patty
Potato
Broccoli
Mixed Green Salad
Dressing
Medium Apple
Cup of Milk

The menus in this chapter are not designed to show how delightfully varied food after fifty can be, even for live-alones. That set of menus is on pages 86-123, with recipes to match on pages 190-206. The menus in this chapter are given simply to illustrate eating feel-better food in threes, or to show amounts required for good nutrition.

Measure for Measure

When Mrs. Shell first told people at the Feel-Better Group the kinds of foods needed at three daily meals to feel better, there was a chorus of protests. "But I could never eat all that food in a day. Never!" "No way!" You may be saying the same thing. But hold on. At the next session of the Feel-Better Group, each food in three sample meals for a day was laid out on a table, as given in the menus above.

Think in Threes • 33

There were gasps of surprise. "Are those all the prunes I need? Just that little bit?" "Is that all the broccoli at dinner?" "What a small serving of meat! I must eat twice that much!"

And that proved to be a big part of the trouble. People were eating such big servings of meat that they had no room for the other good things that are needed to make a real meal.

Here is the actual size serving of the cooked beef patty in our sample dinner menu. It may look small but it gives all the protein needed for an average person over fifty at a main meal.

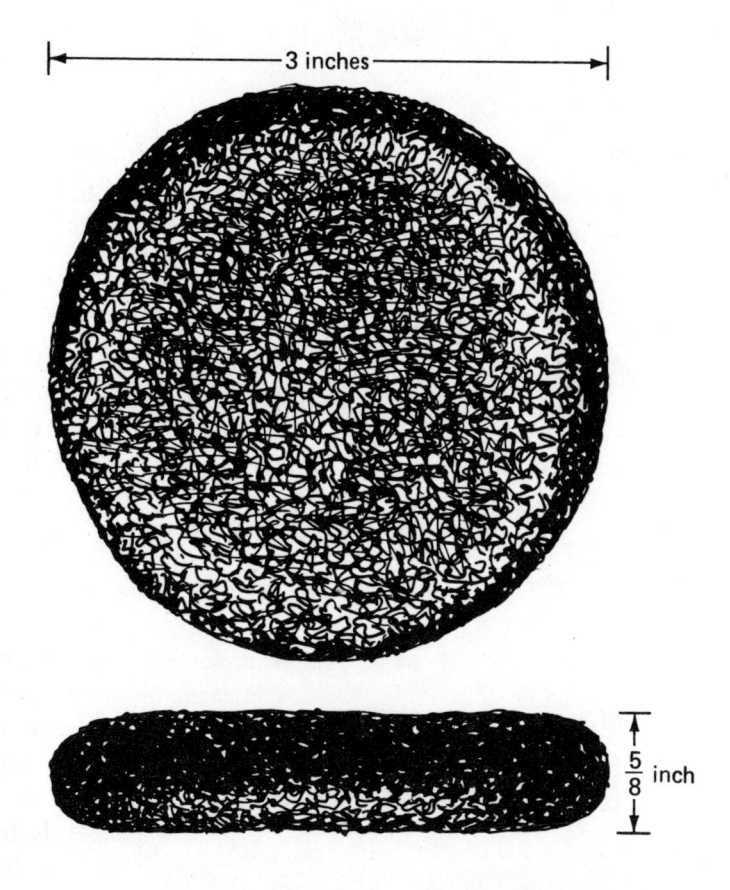

And here's the amount for ham:

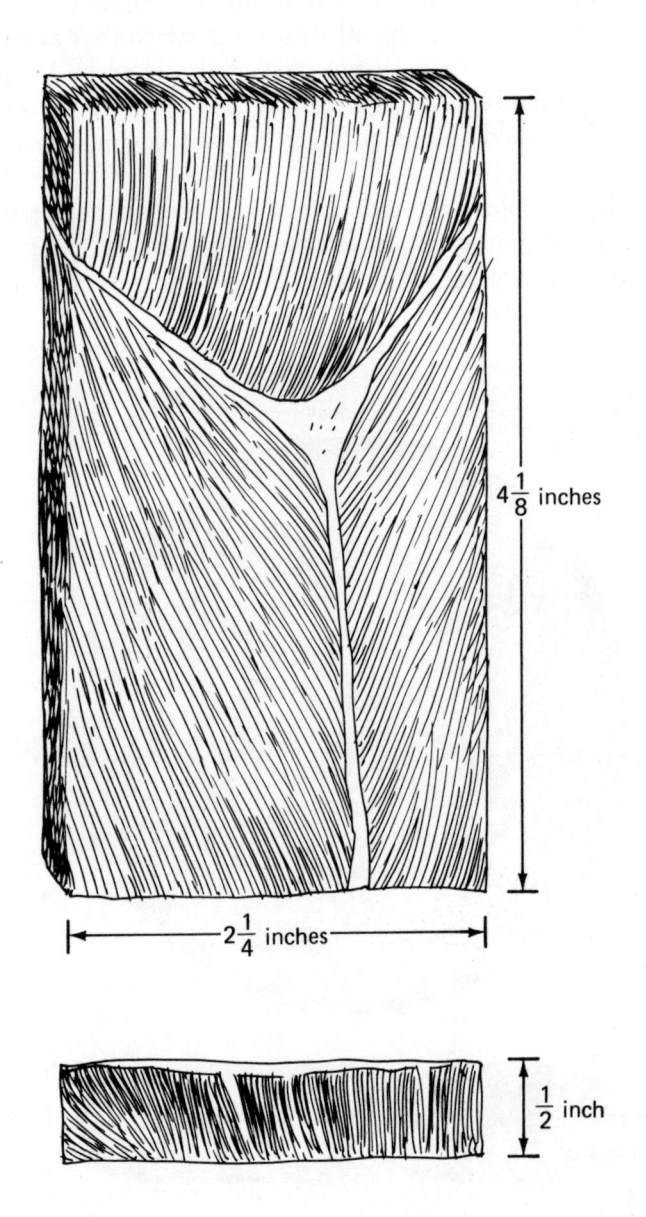

$4\frac{1}{8}$ inches

$2\frac{1}{4}$ inches

$\frac{1}{2}$ inch

And here is how much is needed when steak is served:

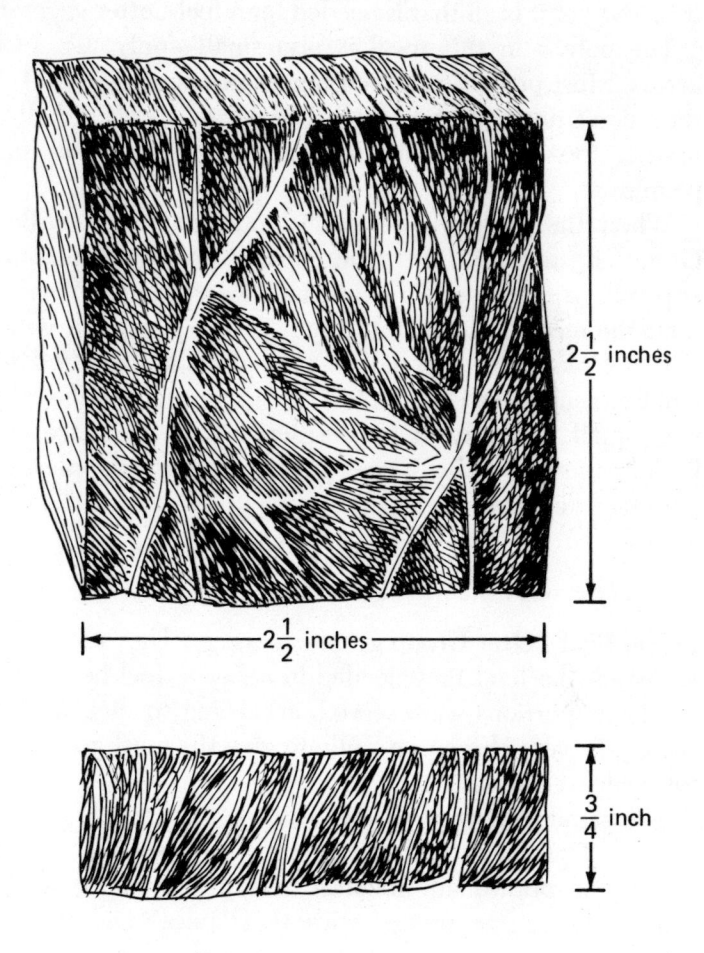

$2\frac{1}{2}$ inches

$2\frac{1}{2}$ inches

$\frac{3}{4}$ inch

Now referring back to the dinner menu again, how about the broccoli? A half-cup is an ample serving to get the benefit of the good things in broccoli. Try this little test. Take a measuring cup, the kind used for cooking, with measurements printed on the side—half-cup, quarter-cup, etc. Put some cooked broccoli, or other vegetable, in the cup to the half-cup mark. You may be amazed at what a small portion it is, and yet it is all that is needed for a feel-better vegetable.

The potato in this meal is also small—only 2½ inches across. Most people eat much bigger potatoes than that, but they don't need to after fifty. The salad is only a half-cup serving too—a doll's portion compared with what many people eat.

When the milk was measured out for the Feel-Better Group, it surprised everyone. It was only one measuring cup full, or 8 ounces. Try this, too, for yourself. When you pour the measured amount of milk into a glass, you will see that it looks more like half a glass of milk compared with what is usually served. As for the apple, people thought it very small. Actually, it is considered a medium-size apple by nutritionists—2¾ inches across, or three apples to a pound of this size.

They Got the Message

The Feel-Better Group got the message. They really *could* easily eat the food they needed in a day to feel better if the right size portions were served, according to their age, and the foods were chosen carefully to give the most good things for the least calories.

The same idea goes all the way through this first day of menus. The feel-better members were amazed that the serving of prunes at breakfast was just a half-cup—only three average-size prunes with their juice. Did you ever measure an ounce of ready-to-eat cereal—the serving recommended on the package? Feel-better people did, and they found that most of them had been eating a lot more in a bowl. The 1-ounce serving averages only one measuring cup full: it's light, bulky stuff that takes up a lot of room.

Here's a word of caution. There are some people who need more food than the above servings because of their

Think in Threes • 37

size or activity, and a few people may need less. A big, tall person needs slightly more than these amounts. Someone smaller who isn't very active needs slightly less. It's very easy to increase or decrease the amounts of food a little to fit your size and degree of activity.

And now for another sample day of "eating in threes" to feel better:

	Amounts
Breakfast	
Feel-Better Breakfast in a Drink	1¼ to 1½ cups
Toast	1 slice
Lunch	
Peanut Butter	3 *level* tablespoons
Sandwich on Whole Wheat Bread	2 slices
Celery and Carrot Sticks	6 to 8 thin sticks about 3 inches long
Ice Cream	½ cup
with Peaches	¼ cup
Milk	½ to 1 cup
Dinner	
Fresh Pork	3 ounces, cooked
Spinach or Kale	½ cup
Potato	2½ inches across
Mixed Vegetable Salad	½ cup
Bread	1 slice
Fresh Fruit	1 piece
Coffee or Tea with Milk	

People are almost sure to have room for this food when it's served in portions right for their age. However, if it proves to be too much, here's another plan.

Mini-Meal Five-a-Day Plan to Feel Better

Some older people do better with five small meals rather than the usual three. The food does just as much good eaten at smaller meals more often, just so long as the total intake is the same for the nutrients the body needs.

Here are the same basic menus as first given, now divided into five small meals with the same good food value.

A Day of Feel-Better Food in Fives

Breakfast
Prunes
Wheat Flakes or
Farina with Milk

Mid-Morning Snack
Toast and Spread
Cup of Milk
Apple

Lunch
Vegetable Soup
Cheese Sandwich

Mid-Afternoon or Evening Snack
Sliced Banana or Peaches
with Milk

Dinner
Beef Patty
Broccoli
Potato
Mixed Green Salad
Beverage

Once you become familiar with the kinds of foods needed every day, you can shuffle them like a deck of cards, and come up with a winning hand every time.

7
The Handy Food Finder

To THE NUTRITIONIST who has studied the matter, each person's body is a miracle with marvelous workings inside. When we don't eat right, we mess up the miracle.

The nutrients in food, such as protein and vitamins, all have special jobs to do in the body to keep it running well. When the body gets all the nutrients it needs, its chemical actions are likely to spin along like a fine-tuned motor. They interact in harmony to keep a person walking, talking, thinking, working, and loving.

Here is a mini-encyclopedia of the nutrients in nontechnical language. It gives the essentials of the major nutrients needed, as far as science knows at this time.

The food nutrients are given in terms of the kind of work they do in the body. They are listed one by one for your convenience so that you can see what each one does, and where it is found. Actually, nutrients do not occur alone in foods. One food usually has several nutrients. In the body, they do their job sometimes separately, sometimes together with one another. The nutrients are given here individually only to identify each one. In feel-better meals, several foods are eaten at once, and all their several nutrients work together for good health.

The figures given here meet the needs of both men and women of fifty years and over. Women may need slightly less of a limited number of the nutrients. However, the guidelines apply to both sexes in most cases.

The foods that are highest in each nutrient are given. This makes it easier to plan feel-better meals, and to choose foods that are the cheapest sources of the nutrient in the market at any season of the year. This saves a lot of money.

Meet the Nutrients

Nutrition is a continuing search for knowledge. Here are the main kinds of nutrients known at this time:

Protein
Fats
Carbohydrates
Vitamins
Minerals
Water

Does that surprise—water a nutrient? It's amazing what a lot of water does in the body, as will soon be found.

Here are the nutrients arranged according to what work they do in the body:

1. Nutrients that build and repair muscles, nerves, brain, bones, teeth and blood
    Protein
    Minerals
    Water

2. Nutrients that give off heat and energy (calories)
    Carbohydrates
    Fats
    Proteins

3. Nutrients that regulate the body
    Water
    Minerals
    Vitamins
    Cellulose (a carbohydrate also known as fiber or roughage)

As you see, some nutrients perform in more than one way in the body, and therefore occur in more than one group.

Protein

Every cell in your body is made of protein. That's how important it is to life—your life. It is essential for good health and vitality. Yet few people know how protein works in the body.

When foods that contain protein are eaten, the food is digested, and the proteins are broken down by the body into amino acids. These are sometimes called building blocks because of the way the body uses them. The amino acids are absorbed into the blood and carried to all the different tissues of the body. Here a remarkable thing happens. Each kind of tissue takes and uses the type of amino acid required to build its own protein, needed for its special purpose in the body. Other amino acids are broken down and changed into fat, which is either used for energy or is stored.

The Three Types of Protein

So that protein foods can be better understood, nutritionists divide them into three kinds: complete protein, partially complete protein, and incomplete protein.

Complete protein has all the essential amino acids in the right amounts and proportions to support growth and maintain life. This kind of protein is found in animal foods: eggs, cheese, meat, milk, fish, chicken.

Partially complete protein sustains life but not growth, if it is the only protein present in the diet. It is found in plant foods: all grains, legumes, fruits, vegetables, nuts.

Incomplete protein neither supports growth nor maintains life because it does not have one or more of the essential amino acids. An example of an incomplete protein food is unflavored or flavored gelatine.

Generally, proteins are called only complete and incomplete, in which case partially complete and incomplete proteins are combined in one group. Amino acids in proteins may also be termed essential or nonessential. Essential amino acids are those that cannot be made in the body. They must come ready-made in the foods we eat. Nonessential amino acids are those made by the body from other nutrients or from essential amino acids in food.

Work That Protein Does in the Body

A good diet must include protein foods because the body needs protein to do all these important jobs:

1. In a normal body, the bone, muscle, nerve, brain, and blood tissues break down constantly and must be replaced daily. Protein is absolutely essential to do this work. We tend to think of new tissue as being needed only by growing children, but this is a need as long as life lasts. People over fifty need protein for this replacement, too, though on a smaller scale than young children.

2. In healthy bodies, the outer skin flakes and scales off constantly. It takes protein to replace it.

3. Protein is needed for the continuing growth and health of hair and nails.

4. Protein plus iron makes the hemoglobin in the blood cells. Hemoglobin carries the breathed-in oxygen from the lungs to the tissues, and then takes away the carbon dioxide from the tissues to the lungs to breathe it out into the air.

5. Enzymes and many hormones are made of protein. They play an important part in the burning of food by the body—called metabolism. When the food burns, it releases energy, or calories, in the body. Enzymes also control the speed of the body's chemical reactions.

6. The body's gamma globulins are made of proteins. They are antibodies that destroy bacteria, viruses, and germs.

Sometimes they are used by the body for short-term or permanent immunity to some diseases.

7. Proteins act as buffers to keep the blood in a slightly alkaline condition, needed for good health.

8. Proteins play a part in controlling the movement of fluids (water balance) in and out of the cells. When this does not work well, edema and other conditions sometimes develop. In edema, the cells hold in fluids, and the tissues become puffy and swollen. This is a common cause of swollen ankles, often suffered by older people.

9. Proteins are used by the body for energy needs (calories) when there are too few carbohydrates and fats in the diet. This is not desirable because the protein which should be used for building and replacing tissues is used in part instead for energy.

Now it can be seen why people whose diets are short in protein foods cannot possibly feel their best. There are so many important workings of the body that depend upon protein, that the body cannot be expected to work well without it.

How Does the Body Show It Is Not Getting Enough Protein?

A shortage of protein foods in the diet is shown in so many ways, it is hard to list them all. Just a few signs are listlessness, lack of vitality, a tired feeling. Other problems caused by a protein shortage are edema, as already mentioned; poor use of foods by the body; wasting of muscle tissue; diarrhea; liver failure, and others. Because the symptoms are so hard to identify, many people feel they are getting along on a diet low in protein foods. Don't take a chance. People who eat the recommended amounts of protein foods daily will be pleased with how much better they feel.

Our Spanish friends often say: "*Respeto! Respeto!*" meaning "Have respect!" That's a good way to think of protein foods.

Protein and Vegetarian Diets

It is important for everyone to be careful to improve the quality of incomplete protein foods by eating some complete protein foods along with them. Simple and easy ways are to eat dishes like macaroni and cheese, cereal with milk, and vegetables with eggs.

Taking care to include more than one protein food in a meal becomes especially important in a vegetarian diet, where only plant foods are eaten. A complete protein meal can be created with a mixture of two or more incomplete or partially complete protein foods that together give the right amounts of amino acids in the right proportions. This is called supplementation or complementarity. It is the secret of good plant vegetarian diets but it takes a lot of knowledge and constant attention to do it right. Plant vegetarians need a vitamin B_{12} supplement because this vitamin is not found in plant foods, and the body cannot work well without it. See Vitamin B_{12}, page 72. Many doctors are now also recommending a zinc supplement.

Vegetarians who eat plant foods plus milk, cheese, and eggs are called lacto-ovo-vegetarians. Eating both plant and animal foods provides complete protein. There is vitamin B_{12} in complete protein foods, calcium in milk, and both iron and zinc in eggs. With careful planning, it is possible to be well-fed on this diet without supplements.

For those who are on vegetarian diets, and are interested in more facts, check with your doctor, or with your library for additional information.

Protein Foods

Most people find they feel better when protein foods make up from 10 percent to 15 percent of their diet. Another way

The Handy Food Finder • 45

of putting it is to say that a diet in which 15 percent of the calories come from protein foods is considered high in protein.

The first group of food portions that follows provides two-thirds of the complete protein needed daily by those over fifty, according to the U.S. Recommended Daily Allowances, but you do not need to eat this entire amount at one meal. In fact, it would be better to have a 2-ounce portion (cooked) of protein food at one meal, and use the other ounce at another meal.

3-Ounce Portions That Give about ⅔ of USRDA of Protein (Complete)

cooked lean chuck beef, flank steak, lean plate beef, lean beef rib roast, lean rump, round steak, lean club, lean porterhouse or T-bone, lean sirloin steak, lean leg lamb, lean fresh-cooked ham, lean baked loin pork roast, stewed domesticated rabbit, veal (medium fat) roast, dark or light meat of chicken (without skin), lean beef heart, kidney, calf or pork liver, broiled cod, baked flounder, tuna in oil (drained)

3-Ounce Portions That Give about ½ of USRDA of Protein (Complete)

lean and fat chuck beef, cooked fresh corned beef, regular and lean ground beef, lean and fat beef rib roast, lean and fat rump, lean and fat leg of lamb, lean and fat cured ham, lean and fat fresh cooked ham, lean and fat baked loin of pork, beef liver, chicken livers, baked blue fish, broiled halibut, boiled shrimp.

Portions That Combine Complete and Incomplete Protein to Give about ½ of USRDA

1 cup of creamed dried chipped beef, 1 cup of Welsh rarebit, 1 cup of homemade recipe for enriched spaghetti and meatballs, 1 cup of chili con carne with beans

Portions That Give about ⅓ of USRDA of Protein (Complete)

½ cup of (pressed down) creamed cottage cheese, 3 ounces of lean and fat club, porterhouse or T-bone steak, steamed cooked crabmeat, cooked (northern) lobster, fried ocean perch, oven-steamed rockfish, canned salmon or 2 ounces of smoked salmon, 1 cup baked custard

Portions That Give about ⅓ of USRDA of Protein (Incomplete)

When using the following foods to meet part of the protein requirement for the day, remember to combine them with some complete protein foods to improve the quality of the incomplete protein.

¾ cup of cooked (dry) soybeans, 1 cup of cooked, drained (dry) Great Northern beans, 1 cup navy, lima, or red kidney beans, 1 cup of cooked whole (dry) lentils, 1 cup cooked (dry) split peas, 4 tablespoons (level) peanut butter

Approximate Amount of Incomplete Protein in Some Popular Foods When Not Eaten in Combination with Complete Protein Foods

1 ounce of ready-to-eat cereal	4%
1 cup of cooked oatmeal	9%
1 cup of cooked brown rice	9%
1 cup of cooked enriched rice	7%
1 cup of cooked enriched noodles	11%
1 cup of al dente enriched spaghetti	11%
1 boiled potato (2½ inches in diameter)	4%
½ cup of cooked carrots	2%

Fats

Fats have a poor reputation with people today. Many may wonder if they need fats at all in the diet, or they may have been avoiding them. The fact is that everyone needs some fats because they play an important part in good health. The fat we eat should be kept to a moderate amount, and some polyunsaturated fats and oils should be included.

Fats are a very complicated subject. There are three kinds of fats—saturated, monounsaturated, and polyunsaturated. Each type of fat is made up of three units of fatty acid and glycerol. The fatty acid part of the fat is like a necklace made up of a chain of beads. These beads are called carbon.

In saturated fats, the carbon beads each have two hydrogen beads attached, and at one end of the necklace there is a cluster of hydrogen, oxygen, and carbon. In monounsaturated fats, hydrogen beads are missing from one of the carbon beads in the chain. In polyunsaturated fats, the hydrogen is missing from two or more beads in the chain. Lard is an example of a saturated fat. Olive oil is a monounsaturated fat, and safflower oil is a polyunsaturated fat.

One reason why people are confused is that they do not understand that saturated, monounsaturated, and polyunsaturated fats (all three kinds) are found in every type of fat in varying amounts and proportions.

Take margarine as an example. Some people are puzzled when they read a margarine label and discover that the product contains about 36 percent polyunsaturated fat, 23 percent saturated, and the remainder monounsaturated. Other margarines are manufactured to give a range of polyunsaturated fat that may be as high as 60 percent. These differences depend upon the type of fats used and the fact that to give margarine a solid form, it may be treated in such a way that part of the polyunsaturated fat becomes saturated.

These differences cause no serious problem, but they do cause confusion. The important thing is to learn how to tell which fat is which, how to use them in the diet, how much to use, and how to avoid the misunderstandings created by words that have no real meaning for consumers.

Saturated Fats

The saturated fats are mostly of animal origin, and they are usually solid in form. They include fats from meat, egg yolk, cheese, milk, butter, variety meats such as kidney and liver, and lard. Coconut oil is a vegetable source of saturated fat.

Unsaturated Fats

The unsaturated, or polyunsaturated, fats are oils made from corn, cottonseed, wheat germ, safflower, peanuts, soybeans, sesame, etc. These oils are used most commonly to make margarine, mayonnaise, and salad dressings. However, there may be other ingredients in these products that contain saturated fats. Mayonnaise, for instance, in addition to oil, is made with egg yolk, a source of saturated fat.

"Hidden" Fats

People in the Feel-Better Group often told us: "I don't eat any fat." We discovered that this meant they weren't eating fats that they could see—or visible fats, as nutritionists call them.

Hidden fats are found in meat, fish such as mackerel and shad, duck, avocado, nuts, whole milk, cream, ice cream, chocolate, most cheeses, peanut butter, and baked goods such as pies, cakes, cookies, and doughnuts. There are small amounts of hidden fats in other foods, too. Many people overlook completely this kind of fat in their diets.

Mayonnaise and salad dressings contain about 80 percent fat. Chocolate and peanut butter are about 50 percent fat. Few people realize that. Cooked pork sausage has about 45 percent fat. Baked goods such as pies, cookies, etc., range from 10 percent to 25 percent fat, and ice cream ranges from 10 percent to 15 percent.

Though fats are important in the diet, people have to be careful not to get too much of them, especially in the form of hidden fats such as peanut butter, chocolate, etc.

Work That Fat Does in the Body

Fats play many roles in the smooth working of the body. They supply concentrated sources of energy, or calories.

They form a protective layer under the skin that helps prevent loss of heat. Ever notice how thin people often complain about the cold?

Fats and oils carry the fat-soluble vitamins such as vitamins A, D, E, and K, and they aid in the absorption of these vitamins by the body.

Fats form a protective cushion, like shock absorbers, around the body's vital organs, and they are needed to form part of every cell structure, to serve as an energy reserve that can be used in time of stress or illness, and to spare protein for body-building and repair rather than for energy use.

Fats supply the essential fatty acids such as linoleic acid which the body cannot make from other nutrients in foods. The body must obtain these fatty acids ready-made in the foods we eat. Fortunately, linoleic acid is found in many oils that come from plants such as corn, cottonseed, soybean, safflower, etc.

Essential fatty acids seem to play a role in the regulation of cholesterol metabolism as well as helping to promote healthy skin and prevent certain types of eczema, dermatitis, and other skin disorders.

It's easy to see why fats in the proper amounts are an important part of the feel-better diet.

Amounts of Fat for After-Fifty Eaters

For persons over fifty (unless restricted by a doctor), three to four *small* portions of visible fat are recommended along with the hidden fat in foods, such as lean meat and dairy products, in amounts suggested in the feel-better diet and the Daily Food Guide, page 79.

What is a small portion? It's any of the following:

1½ teaspoons	butter, margarine, vegetable oil, or other clear (liquid) fat
2 level tablespoons	light or sour cream
1 level tablespoon	French dressing

As for the essential fatty acids, the Food and Nutrition Board of the National Research Council recommends that they be used in an amount equal to one to two percent of the total calorie intake. For most people, this is met easily in the diet by including daily two to three teaspoons of a polyunsaturated oil made from corn, safflower, or the other plant sources as mentioned above.

The Fats Controversy

When fats were discussed in the Feel-Better Group, confusion and fear were expressed in reaction to the controversy about the relationship of dietary fats and cholesterol to atherosclerosis, a coronary heart disease in which cholesterol and other fatty substances are deposited on the inner walls of the arteries.

The confusion was caused by three things: the less than clear information from so-called experts; early advertising claims concerning polyunsaturates; differing opinions from scientists as to the specific role played by foods and nutrients, especially fats, in increasing or decreasing the risk of atherosclerosis.

The fact is that diet is only one of many factors associated with the development of atherosclerosis and increased risk of coronary heart disease. Other risk factors are metabolic diseases such as diabetes, stress, cigarette smoking, lack of exercise, heredity, obesity, high blood pressure, and more than normal amounts of blood lipids.

The greatest misunderstanding on the part of the public concerns blood lipids. These include triglycerides, fatty acids, cholesterol, and other fatlike substances. Cholesterol has been discussed so much as playing a bad role in the body, it may come as a shock to many people to learn that it also does many good things for the body. Cholesterol is an important part of all animal tissues and cells, including our own. Both the sex glands and the adrenal gland use cholesterol to make certain hormones. The liver converts cholesterol into bile acids which help digest foods properly. It also surprises people to discover that even if foods containing cholesterol were not eaten, the body makes cholesterol on its own.

People with atherosclerosis usually have a higher blood cholesterol level than people without it. People with high cholesterol levels are known to develop this disease more often than those with normal levels. To date, studies have not shown conclusively that restricting dietary cholesterol in the general population reduces the frequency of atherosclerosis.

However, scientists agree that a balanced diet suitable for a person's age and activity, keeping to desirable weight, moderation in the total amount of fat, and variety in the kinds of fat or fatty acids in the diet are important to health at every age.

Fats and the Feel-Better Diet

If you are eating large amounts of fat, cut down. You have lots of company! About 45 percent of the calories in the average American diet comes from fat. People would feel better if they cut this back to about 30 percent to 35 percent of their total calorie intake. If animal fat makes up most of your fat intake, cut it back but don't cut it out. Strike a balance between animal fats and the polyunsaturated fats both in your cooking and as table fats.

It is wise to choose lean cuts of meat and to cook them by broiling, baking, or in water, rather than by deep-fat frying. People who eat large amounts of red meat every day could cut back on fat if they eat red meat only once or twice a week, and have chicken, fish, or low-fat cheese such as cottage cheese the other days. The greater variety adds more interest to meals, too.

If you use large amounts of cream, butter, sour cream, etc., cut back to reasonable amounts. People who use coffee creamer substitute will find by reading labels that most of these products are made with coconut or palm oil, which are high food sources of cholesterol.

It's wise, too, to cut back on amounts of bacon, sausage, frankfurters, and other meats with high fat content.

Special Note on Mineral Oil

Did you know that mineral oil is not a food fat? It is not made from plants but is a by-product of petroleum. Mineral oil is not digested by the body. It just passes through as part of the feces, or stools. Because this oil does not have calories, some people use it to make low-calorie salad dressings. This is not a good idea because mineral oil dissolves fat-soluble vitamins so that the body cannot use them. Also, when mineral oil is used as a laxative, it carries important nutrients through the body as waste before they can be used. For these reasons, mineral oil is no longer allowed in the making of commercial salad dressings.

Carbohydrates

Recently, carbohydrate foods went out of style with the public in the big fad for reducing diets. People who go on meat and salad reducing diets often end up telling the doctor that their energy is so low they can hardly drag themselves around. They feel as if they haven't the strength to lift a finger. The doctor tells them to put carbohydrate foods back in their diet to give them the energy they need, and never to limit their diet to just two or three foods.

There are three main forms of carbohydrates:

Starches
Sugars
Celluloses (fiber)

The starches and sugars in carbohydrates are the major sources of energy (calories) for humans.

The celluloses furnish bulk, which is essential in the diet for the body to work well.

Why the Body Needs Carbohydrates

The body has an amazing ability to break down sugars and starches to make glucose, or blood sugar, which it must have to work. Glucose is used by the cells to furnish energy to the body and to help support body activity.

Carbohydrates, once they are digested, are absorbed into the blood through the intestine, and then go to the liver to be changed mainly into glucose and glycogen. The glycogen is stored in the body while the glucose remains in the blood to be used by the cells.

Other jobs that carbohydrates do in the body are to spare proteins by supplying the energy needed for the body's work, to help the body to use fats more efficiently, and to provide the bulk, that is, food fiber or roughage, necessary to stimulate the intestinal muscle movement that prevents constipation.

Good Sources of Starch

Grains such as wheat, oats, corn, rice
Products made from grains such as breads, breakfast cereals, flours, macaroni, spaghetti, noodles, grits
Vegetables such as potatoes, sweet potatoes
Legumes such as dry beans and peas

These carbohydrate foods, in addition to giving energy, also furnish incomplete protein, vitamins, minerals, and fiber.

Concentrated Sources of Sugar

Cane and beet sugar
Jellies and jams
Most candies and other sweets
Honey, molasses and syrups

These carbohydrate foods should be limited in the diet because they are high in calories and very low, or altogether lacking, in nutrients. Concentrated sweets may irritate the gastrointestinal tract when eaten in large amounts. They also dull the appetite for foods high in nutrition. To satisfy the need for concentrated sweets, use fresh or dried fruits. Restrict soft drinks, which are diluted, flavored syrups.

Good Sources of Cellulose (Fiber)

Fruits
Vegetables
Whole grain cereals

Although celluloses are not digested by the body, they furnish important bulk, and are accompanied in the above foods by essential nutrients.

How Much Carbohydrate Is Needed?

Most nutritionists feel that carbohydrates should make up about 50 percent to 55 percent of the calories in the day's meals. Special skill in combining carbohydrates (supplementation) makes it possible to increase the carbohydrate foods to a larger percentage of the diet without going short on protein.

Because carbohydrate needs in the diet are expressed by nutritionists in percentages of total calorie needs, portions of these foods cannot be given in ounces and cupfuls. However, in the Daily Food Guide, page 79, you will find recommended servings of carbohydrate foods along with many others. Note the carbohydrate foods given above as highest sources; then be sure to eat them in the amounts given in the Daily Food Guide.

Our menus provide plenty of carbohydrate foods for a feel-better diet, and these needs are also carefully considered in our recipes.

The Handy Food Finder • 55

Despite what you may have heard, the starch carbohydrate foods will never make you fat if eaten in the correct amounts each day. A typical day's meals might include carbohydrate in the form of two slices of bread, a bowl of cereal, and a starchy vegetable, such as a small potato. That won't make you fat and that's a promise—the scientific truth. For further detail, see chapter 10, "Never Have To Diet Again."

Fiber

Food fiber, also called roughage or cellulose, provides bulk, which stimulates the normal action of the intestinal tract to remove waste. Food fiber also absorbs many times its weight in water. This makes softer stools which are easier to pass out of the body.

The daily need for fiber in the diet is met easily by including two fruits, two vegetables, and two servings of whole grain cereals in each day's total meals. The estimated need for fiber is 4 to 7 milligrams. Here for your reference we include a table of the fiber content of some common foods.

Fiber Content of Food

Food	Fiber Content
Apple, unpeeled (medium)	1.5 mg
Squash, winter, cooked, ½ cup	1.4 mg
Broccoli, chopped, cooked, ½ cup	1.2 mg
Corn on cob, cooked (1 ear)	1.0 mg
Strawberries, ½ cup	1.0 mg
Soybeans, cooked, ½ cup	1.0 mg
Banana, 1 medium	0.9 mg
Bread, whole wheat, 2 slices	0.9 mg
Carrots, cooked, ½ cup	0.7 mg
Beans, green, cooked, ½ cup	0.6 mg
Cabbage, cooked, ½ cup	0.6 mg
Potato, baked in skin, medium	0.6 mg
Squash, summer, cooked, ½ cup	0.6 mg
Bulgur, wheat, cooked, ½ cup	0.5 mg

Food	Fiber Content
Chard, Swiss, cooked, ½ cup	0.5 mg
Peas, cooked, ½ cup	0.5 mg
Spinach, cooked, ½ cup	0.5 mg
Lettuce, romaine, 2 leaves	0.4 mg
Potatoes, mashed, ½ cup	0.4 mg
Cabbage, raw, shredded, ½ cup	0.3 mg
Crackers, graham, 4	0.3 mg
Lettuce, ⅛ head	0.3 mg
Rice, brown, cooked, ½ cup	0.3 mg
Cornflakes, ½ cup	0.2 mg
Rice, white, cooked, ½ cup	0.1 mg
Noodles or macaroni, cooked, ½ cup	0.1 mg
*Bran (sugar and malt), ⅓ cup	1.6 mg
*Bran flakes (40% bran), 1 cup	1.3 mg
Wheat flakes (unsweetened), 1 cup	0.5 mg
Wheat germ, 1 tablespoon	0.1 mg
Wheat, shredded, 1 ounce	0.6 mg
Beans, lima, canned, ½ cup	1.5 mg
Pear, raw with skin, 1 medium	2.0 mg
Kale, cooked, ½ cup	0.7 mg

* Check labels of bran products for fiber content of specific brands.

Special Statement on Bran

Too liberal use of bran, as well as of other foods eaten for roughage, can cause digestive disturbances in some people. For those who suffer from an "irritable colon," peptic ulcer, or other gastrointestinal disturbances, the amount of roughage in the diet must be limited.

Water

Yes, water is a nutrient!

When most people think about food, good nutrition, and feeling better, they never think of water as a nutrient. Water is absolutely essential to life. A person can live longer without food than without water, or other liquid. One can live without food for weeks but only for a few days without water.

Besides the water one drinks, one gets water from foods such as vegetables, fruits, meats, from soups, milk, and juices. As the body burns food, water is released.

Work That Water Does in the Body

Water regulates body temperature.

It is a part of all body fluids, such as blood, secretions, and excretions. It carries food materials from one part of the body to another.

It aids digestion by helping to dissolve food. It is essential to good elimination.

How Much Water Is Needed?

For most people, six to eight glasses of water a day, or fluids such as juice, etc., are more than adequate. If you really want to feel better, start your day by drinking a glass or two of water immediately after getting out of bed. If one does not get enough water, even though all the other elements of a good diet are provided, the body cannot work as well. It takes a regular and generous intake of water for all the jobs that the body needs to do. People who have problems with water retention may have to limit their intake, according to a doctor's instructions.

Vitamins

Vitamins are essential to life. They play one of the most vital roles in the body. They also help promote normal growth of different kinds of tissues, take part in the release of energy from food, and are essential to the proper working of nerves and tissues.

It is important to know that vitamins not only work alone but also with one another, and with other nutrients. The lack of one vitamin often affects the requirements and the working of the others.

Most experts feel that there are vitamins still to be discovered. We can act only on the knowledge that we have so far. But this can help us to feel a lot better. Remember, though, the vitamin story is a continuing one of research and discovery.

Let's look at some of the things that we do know about vitamins and the way they work in the body to help people to feel better.

Fat-Soluble Vitamins

Vitamins A, D, K, and E are fat soluble. They dissolve in fat, and fats carry the vitamins throughout the body to do their work. When you cook fat-soluble-vitamin foods in fat, it is important to eat the fat along with the food. Otherwise you will be throwing the vitamins away.

Vitamin A

What does this vitamin do in the body?

It promotes normal growth and tissue repair. It maintains healthy eyes and normal vision. The eye is one of the first parts of the body to show the ill effects of a diet low in vitamin A. This is one of the causes of night blindness. In a very serious lack of vitamin A in the diet, the tear glands may also be affected. This can cause blindness.

Vitamin A also keeps the lining (mucous membrane) wet inside the mouth, throat, and digestive and urinary tract. Why is this important? When this dries out, one is more likely to get infections such as sinus trouble, sore throat, abscesses in the ears, mouth, or the glands in the mouth. Some older people experience "dry mouth," and a shortage of vitamin A may be one of the causes.

Vitamin A also plays an important part in keeping the bones and teeth healthy.

Signs of Vitamin A Shortage

In children, the signs are retarded growth, faulty bone and tooth development. In adults, the signs are dry, rough scaly skin, infections as mentioned above, night blindness and glare blindness.

Effects of Too Much Vitamin A

Large amounts of vitamin A are toxic. However, vitamin A toxicity is seldom caused by food alone. It usually occurs through taking large doses of vitamin A pills. Be careful about this. It can cause swelling of the feet and ankles, overtiredness, loss of weight, pains that come and go in the shoulders, wrists, and knees. In some people, the skin becomes coarse and breaks open, and there is an itching rash. There is thinning of the hair. There are also pains in the joints caused by bleeding between the bones that can't be seen.

Remember that though vitamin A can cause all these symptoms, they can also be due to other body problems, so check your doctor if you have them.

The Vitamin A Foods

Vitamin A usually comes from animal foods—liver, eggs, etc. However, plant foods such as carrots, sweet potatoes, cantaloupes, etc., have a substance called carotene which the body can make into vitamin A, and it has the same effect.

Portions of Food That Provide All the USRDA of Vitamin A

3 ounces of cooked liver (beef, calf, pork or chicken), ½ cup of cooked carrots, sweet potatoes, spinach, pumpkin, collards, peas and carrots, dandelion greens, turnip greens, kale, mixed vegetables, mustard greens, garden cress, winter squash, or other very dark green leafy vegetable, also dark orange fruit such as ½ raw mango (about ⅓ lb.), or ½ a raw cantaloupe (5-inch diameter)

Portions of Food That Give about ½ to ¾ of the USRDA of Vitamin A

½ cup of cooked broccoli, canned apricots, or raw chopped spinach, 1 raw red pepper, 3 fresh apricots, 1 cup of canned plums, 6 to 8 raw carrot strips (2½ to 3 inches long), 1 cup cubed raw papaya, 1 cup cooked tomatoes, 4 x 8-inch wedge watermelon, ⅙ of 9-inch pumpkin or sweet potato pie, 1 cup of vegetable beef or vegetarian vegetable soup

Vitamin A is found in less concentrated amounts in many foods besides those listed above. This vitamin is found in milk, butter or margarine, cream, Cheddar or American cheese, ice cream and recipes made with milk. As these foods are eaten in meals, they add an important amount of vitamin A to the body's total intake. For example, when the meals for any one day include two glasses of milk, one egg, 1 tablespoon butter or margarine, the vitamin A adds up to about one-third the Recommended Daily Allowance. Another day of meals might include one glass of milk, 1 ounce of Cheddar cheese and a half-cup of baked custard. This would give one-fourth the Recommended Daily Allowance of vitamin A.

How to Keep Vitamin A in Foods

Vitamin A is destroyed by exposure to air and light. There is also a gradual loss when vitamin A foods are exposed to high, dry temperature. To avoid this, store vitamin A foods in a cool, dark place, or in the refrigerator. Vitamin A is stable to heat and usual cooking methods. But don't forget that it is soluble in fat. When you cook vitamin A foods in fat, eat the fat along with the food. Otherwise, you throw vitamin A away.

Vitamin D

Vitamin D is a fat-soluble vitamin that is essential for growth and development, and for the upkeep of the bones and teeth. It aids in the best use of calcium and phosphorus by the body.

Vitamin D is produced by the action of direct sunlight on the skin. The sunlight that most people are usually exposed to is filtered through glass, clothing, and the atmosphere, and this cannot be depended upon for the vitamin D needed by the body. Few foods contain much vitamin D. For these reasons, most milk in the stores has been fortified with vitamin D. Fortified milk is the main source of this vitamin for most people.

Here is a shopping caution. In the past year, some milk has been sold at a cheaper price because it is not fortified with Vitamin D. It is strongly advisable to buy either fluid whole milk or nonfat dry milk, with vitamin D added. Check labels to be sure.

Vitamin D Foods

Fish liver oils
Vitamin D milk
Egg yolk
Liver
Salt-water fish

Signs of a vitamin D shortage are rickets, bow legs, soft bones, and poor teeth. Vitamin D is stable to heat and keeps well under normal conditions.

Vitamin K

Vitamin K is needed by the body to form a substance called prothrombin, which is essential to normal blood clotting. Doctors can detect a shortage of vitamin K in a test which shows a slow blood clotting time. Some people bruise easily when the body is deficient in vitamin K.

Vitamin K is stable to heat and air.

Vitamin K Foods

Cauliflower
Cabbage
Green leafy vegetables
Soybean oil

Recommended servings are not given because vitamin K is widely distributed in small amounts in many foods, and the body itself makes vitamin K.

Vitamin E

The full role of vitamin E in the body is not yet understood. We do know, however, that vitamin E is essential to the structure, building, and working of the cells, particularly in the formation of the blood cells.

Vitamin E Foods

Wheat germ, and germ of other cereals
Peanuts
Corn
Soybeans
Green leafy vegetables
Fruits
Nuts
Vegetable oils
Margarine

Recommended servings are not given for vitamin E because it is so widely distributed in the above foods, and others.

People who suffer from conditions that interfere with the digestion or absorption of fats by the body may require vitamin E supplementation. This should be done under a doctor's care.

A vitamin E shortage is hard to identify because it has no visible effects. It requires a blood test to detect it. Usually, lack of vitamin E results in a mild anemia with abnormal red blood cell breakdown.

Vitamin E is stable to ordinary cooking methods.

Water-Soluble Vitamins

All vitamins, except A, K, D, and E, are water soluble. The water that you cook vitamin-rich foods in will be full of vitamins, so have it with the foods or save it to flavor soups. Many leftovers can be stored in the liquid you cooked them in.

Vitamin C

Although there is still debate on how vitamin C, a water-soluble vitamin, works in the body, it is known that it plays a role in protecting against infections and bacteria. It is also important for maintaining healthy gums and teeth.

Vitamin C helps to make collagen in the body, a protein important in the formation of skin, tendon, bone, and supportive tissue. It helps give strength to blood vessel walls. It affects the formation of hemoglobin and of iron.

Signs of Vitamin C Shortage

A severe shortage of vitamin C in the diet used to show up as scurvy. This disease once killed sailors who were unable to get any vitamin C foods at all on voyages that could last for years. Scurvy is seldom seen today but lack of vitamin C in the diet may show up in delayed healing of wounds and fractures, or after an operation. A deficiency may also show in feelings of weakness, loss of weight, and fleeting pains in the arms and legs which are often mistaken for arthritis pains. A vitamin C shortage can play a part in secondary anemia.

How to Keep Vitamin C in Foods

Vitamin C is the most unstable of all the vitamins in storage and preparation. It is affected by air, heat, and alkaline substances such as baking soda. Never use a copper pot when cooking high vitamin C foods. It destroys the "C."

Vitamin C is also lost by the aging and drying of food, and in the cooking water. Vitamin C dissolves in water. To preserve vitamin C that escapes into cooking water, be sure to serve the liquid as part of a meal rather than pouring it down the drain. Cooking vitamin C foods in a minimum amount of water is important.

Portions of Food That Give All the USRDA of Vitamin C

½ cup of cooked broccoli, collards, Brussels sprouts, green or red pepper, kale or turnip greens, a raw green or red pepper, ½ cup of orange or grapefruit juice, ⅔ cup of raw strawberries, ¼ of (5-inch diameter) raw cantaloupe, ½ cup of orange or grapefruit sections (1 medium orange or ½ of a large grapefruit), 1 cup of tomatoes

Portions of Food That Give 70 to 90 percent of USRDA of Vitamin C

1 cup of canned tangerine, sauerkraut or tomato juice, 1 cup of cooked cabbage, spinach, or rutabaga, 1 cup of shredded green or red cabbage, 1 tomato (3-inch diameter), 1 medium lemon

Portions of Food That Give about ½ of USRDA of Vitamin C

½ cup of cooked asparagus pieces, okra, peas, sauerkraut, turnips, ½ cup of cabbage (common or savoy) raw, finely shredded, or raw coleslaw, 1 cup of raw loganberries, blackberries, or raspberries, watermelon (4 x 8-inch wedge), 1 cup of pineapple juice, medium potato (baked in skin)

B Vitamins

Nature has been very generous with the amounts of vitamins A and C concentrated in particular foods. As you've seen, you can get your entire day's supply of these vitamins in a half-cup serving of one food—orange or grapefruit juice for vitamin C—sweet potatoes or carrots for vitamin A.

It's different with the B vitamins. Very few foods can supply the total daily need for B vitamins by themselves. Instead, these vitamins are found in smaller concentrations in a wide range of foods. Here again, a variety of foods must be eaten to fill the need. You may feel that many single foods which are listed give only a small amount of the B vitamins but they add up to fill the day's needs.

For example, when you include in your diet a good ready-to-eat breakfast cereal and a slice of bread at breakfast, and two slices of bread at lunch, you are meeting about 40 percent of your thiamine needs for the day, even though one slice of bread has only 6 percent or 7 percent of the thiamine needed by a person over fifty. In addition, if you were to add a 3-ounce serving of fresh-cooked pork, you would be getting your thiamine needs for the day. It takes a combination of foods to get your B vitamins, so don't be surprised if the amounts of nutrients per food seem small.

Thiamine, or Vitamin B_1

This vitamin is known as the "morale vitamin" because without it, many people feel washed out, as the saying has it.

Thiamine works in the body to help promote normal appetite and digestion. It is one factor involved in the release of energy from the burning of carbohydrate foods in the body. It is needed for healthy muscle tone within the body. We've all seen people who seem to have a bouncy, lively quality to their skin and their movement. That's good muscle tone. Thiamine is also needed for the proper working of the heart, nerves, and muscle. Remember thiamine is water-soluble, so when you cook in water, be sure to use or save the liquid.

Signs of Thiamine Shortage. People who do not get enough thiamine become irritable, quarrelsome, moody. They are not cooperative with others, and at times suffer from depression. In extreme cases, a thiamine deficiency results in the disease called beriberi. Although this disease is seldom seen, it is sometimes suffered by alcoholics. The symptoms of beriberi are numbness or tingling in toes and feet, ankle stiffness, ankle jerk reflex and cramping pains in the legs, difficulty in walking, and finally paralysis of the legs with wasting of the leg muscles.

Even with a mild thiamine deficiency, there is fatigue, loss of appetite, constipation, labored breathing, nausea. These signs may also be associated with deficiencies of other nutrients.

Remember thiamine is water-soluble, so when you cook thiamine-rich foods in water, serve the liquid as part of the meal. Otherwise, the thiamine is thrown away with the water.

Portion of Food That Gives about ¾ of USRDA of Thiamine

3 ounces of cooked sliced pork loin (lean only)

Portions of Food That Give about ½ of USRDA of Thiamine

3 ounces of cooked sliced pork loin, lean and fat, 2.7 ounces of cooked loin pork chop, lean and fat, 1 cup of ground lean fresh or cured ham or shoulder, 2 ounces of lean loin pork chop

Portions of Food That Give about ⅓ of USRDA of Thiamine

3 ounces of cooked fresh ham, beef kidney, cured ham, spareribs, 1 cup of cooked (dry) cowpeas or soybeans, 1 cup of cooked green peas, 1 ounce of ready-to-eat cereals (check label)

Portions That Give about ¼ of USRDA of Thiamine

3 ounces of cooked pork liver, 1 cup of cooked (dry) navy beans, 1 cup of home made beef pot pie or chicken pot pie

(⅓ of 9-inch pie), 1 cup of cooked, drained fresh lima beans, or 1 cup of peas and carrots

Portions That Give about ⅕ of USRDA of Thiamine

3 ounces of cooked beef heart, beef liver or calf liver, 1 patty (1 ounce) of pork sausage, 1 cup of cooked (dry) Great Northern, lima or red kidney beans, 1 cup of homemade baked macaroni and cheese, canned beans in tomato sauce with pork, homemade spaghetti (enriched) in tomato sauce with cheese, or spaghetti (enriched) in tomato sauce with meatballs, 1 cup of cooked, drained asparagus pieces, collards, okra, sprouted soybean seeds, turnip greens, or mixed vegetables (carrots, corn, peas, green snap beans, lima beans), homemade potato salad with cooked salad dressing, 1 cup fresh orange juice, 1 cup of spoon bread made of white, whole-ground corn meal, 1 hard roll (round or rectangular) made of enriched flour, gingerbread (3 x 3 x 2 inches) made with enriched flour, 1 cup of cooked (hot) enriched macaroni, noodles or spaghetti, ⅙ of a 9-inch pecan pie, 1 cup of homemade bread (enriched) pudding with raisins, 1 cup of split-pea soup, or 3 slices of whole wheat or enriched bread

Portions of Food That Give about 6 to 10 Percent of USRDA of Thiamine

1 cup of skim milk or buttermilk or yogurt, 3 ounces of cooked lean ground beef or lamb, 3 ounces of cooked bass, blue fish or ocean perch, 1 cup of cooked broccoli, cauliflower, carrots, eggplant, kale, mustard greens, parsnips, canned peas, cooked tomatoes, succotash (corn and lima beans), tomato or vegetable juice, 1 bagel (3-inch diameter), 1 baking powder biscuit (2-inch diameter) made with enriched flour, 1 slice of whole grain or enriched bread, 1 muffin (about 2⅜") made with enriched flour, 1 cup of cooked degerminated, enriched grits, 1 cup of bean soup with pork

Nuts such as filberts, almonds, chestnuts, English walnuts, provide additional thiamine when used as a snack or part of a main dish.

Riboflavin, or Vitamin B_2

This is a water-soluble vitamin that helps the cells to use oxygen. It literally assists the cells to breathe and stay alive. It also helps keep the skin, tongue, and lips normal, and prevents scaly, greasy skin around the mouth and nose.

Portions of Food That Give All of USRDA of Riboflavin

3 ounces of cooked beef kidney, 3 ounces cooked pork, beef, calf, or chicken liver

Portion of Food That Gives about ⅔ of USRDA of Riboflavin

3 ounces of cooked lean beef heart

Portions of Food That Give about ⅓ of USRDA of Riboflavin

1 cup of cottage cheese, malted beverage, or baked custard, 1 cup of creamed chipped beef or Welsh rarebit

Portions of Food That Give about ¼ of USRDA of Riboflavin

1 cup of whole or skim milk, buttermilk, soft-serve ice cream or ice milk, yogurt, tapioca cream, cooked lean leg of lamb (diced), cooked lean pork (diced), cooked veal (diced), homemade chicken à la king, homemade macaroni (enriched) and cheese, 1 cup of cooked lean chopped beef, lamb, ham or dark turkey meat, stuffed pepper, home recipe spaghetti (enriched) with meatballs, 1 cup of cooked broccoli, collards or turnip greens, 1-ounce serving ready-to-eat cereal (check label), or 1 cup of spoon bread made with

whole ground corn meal, 1 cup of cream of mushroom soup made with milk

There are many foods which contribute small amounts of riboflavin that add up importantly when used in meals on a regular basis. These foods include Cheddar cheese, whole grain or enriched breads, cooked dried peas and beans, almonds, whole eggs, and many other foods. Each slice of enriched or whole grain bread provides 4 percent of the USRDA for riboflavin.

Niacin

Niacin, along with other vitamins, plays an important part in changing carbohydrate into energy. It is needed for the normal working of both the gastrointestinal tract and the nervous system. Niacin helps the cells to breathe, and it also helps to maintain normal skin.

Without niacin in the diet, pellagra could develop. This is a serious disease which is rarely seen in the United States. However, pellagra is still found in areas where corn and other highly refined grains along with fat make up most of the diet.

3-Ounce Portions of Food that Give All the USRDA of Niacin

cooked liver (pork, calf, beef, or chicken), tuna, cooked rabbit, kidney, light and dark meat of chicken or turkey, swordfish, goose, salmon steak, lean veal, beef heart, halibut, mackerel, or shad

Portions of Food That Give about ¾ of USRDA of Niacin

3 ounces of cooked lean pork or fresh ham, canned salmon, lean beef steak, ground beef, lean lamb, or canned sardines, 1 cup of homemade beef and vegetable stew, corned beef hash, spaghetti (enriched) with cheese

Portions of Food That Give about ½ of USRDA of Niacin

1 ounce of peanuts or 2 tablespoons of peanut butter, 1 cup of homemade chicken and noodles, homemade chow mein, homemade spaghetti (enriched) with meatballs, 1 cup of cooked green peas, 1 ounce of ready-to-eat cereal (check label)

It is interesting that niacin can be produced in the body from the essential amino acid, tryptophan. However, though it is a poor source of niacin, milk is an excellent source of tryptophan. Two glasses of milk provide enough tryptophan to supply about a quarter of the daily need for niacin because the tryptophan produces niacin in the body.

Like the other B vitamins, there are many foods which provide small amounts of niacin. These are important in the diet in their total effect. An example is three slices of whole wheat bread or enriched white bread which give about one-third the niacin needed for the day. The same is true of other enriched bread products, and of enriched rice and pasta products.

Vitamin B_6

Vitamin B_6 does a very special job in the use of protein by the body. It also plays a part in the metabolism of polyunsaturated fats, amino acids, and carbohydrates, and it is involved in the change of tryptophan to niacin.

Here's a dramatic example of how important this vitamin is to the body. During the 1950s, it was found that babies fed exclusively on a liquid formula made by a certain manufacturer were suffering from irritability, muscle-twitching, and even convulsions. Careful study determined that the only change the company had made in manufacturing its formula was to use higher heat in sterilizing than previously. This change destroyed the vitamin B_6 in the formula, and the absence of the vitamin in the babies' diets caused their irritability, twitchiness, and convulsions.

Signs of Vitamin B_6 Shortage. A vitamin B_6 shortage in the diet of adults shows up as weakness, depression, sleepiness, loss of appetite, nausea, and anemia which does not respond to increasing the iron in the diet.

How to Keep Vitamin B_6 in Foods. Vitamin B_6 is destroyed by light and heat. The greatest loss of this vitamin comes in the milling of grains. As Dr. Jean Mayer, the noted nutritionist points out, it is very important to know that about 75 percent of the vitamin B_6 is removed by the milling of white flour. It is not replaced even when flour is enriched. In order to get the amount of this vitamin that is needed, whole grain breads and cereals must be included in the diet.

Vitamin B_6 Foods. The small amount of B_6 needed by the body is easily supplied when there is a variety of foods in the diet. These foods should include:

Meat, fish, and shellfish
Wheat germ
Whole grain breads and cereals
   (important because B_6 is removed in the milling of white flour and not replaced by enrichment)
Cabbage
Potatoes and sweet potatoes
Spinach, as well as most dark green, leafy vegetables
Prunes and raisins
Bananas
Chicken
Dry legumes
Egg yolk
Yeast
Peanuts, walnuts, filberts, and peanut butter

Vitamin B_{12}

This vitamin is essential for the growth and proper working of all body cells, and the development of red blood cells.

It plays a role in the use of fat and carbohydrate, and it is the substance in the liver that may control pernicious anemia.

Signs of a vitamin B_{12} shortage in the diet are like those of the other B vitamins, except for pernicious anemia which is the deficiency symptom most under study.

Special Note for Plant Vegetarians. It is important to know that plant foods do not have vitamin B_{12} and that the body cannot make this vitamin by itself. Without B_{12} in the diet, a serious anemia can develop, which results in listlessness, tiredness, irritability, and other symptoms.

We strongly advise vegetarians who eat only plant foods to ask their doctor for a B_{12} supplement. It would also be wise to take an iron, calcium, and zinc supplement because it is very difficult to meet the body's needs for these minerals on most plant vegetarian diets.

Vitamin B_{12} is destroyed by heat and gradually destroyed by light. Vitamin B_{12} foods include:

Liver
Meat
Whole eggs and egg yolk
Milk
Kidney
Most cheese
Most fish
Shellfish

Folacin

This vitamin is essential for making hemoglobin in the body. It plays a role in amino acid metabolism, and it is needed for the proper development of the red blood cells.

Symptoms of a shortage of folacin are a special type of anemia, tropical sprue, tiredness, and a rundown feeling.

Folacin is destroyed by heat, and also by sunlight if the food stands at room temperature. Folacin foods include:

Dark green leafy vegetables
Liver
Kidney
Dry beans
Peanuts
Wheat germ

Minerals

The body needs minerals to give strength to certain tissues and to help in its many vital workings. Just as with the B vitamins, nature has not concentrated the minerals in any one food, but has spread them throughout practically all.

For instance, you can get your total day's need for iron in an average serving of only a few foods, such as calf or pork liver. There is no serving of food in the amounts normally eaten at a meal that can give you all of the calcium needed by the body for a day.

Calcium

There is more calcium in the body than any other mineral. All but 1 percent of the calcium is found in bones and teeth. The remaining calcium, though small in amount, does important jobs in the body. Besides keeping bones and teeth strong and healthy, calcium is one of the essential factors for blood clotting in blood plasma, it affects muscle tone and movement, and is needed for normal nerve functioning. Together with other minerals, calcium aids in normal, rhythmic contraction and relaxation of the heart muscle. Blood calcium level in the body is related to the working of a gland and hormone which regulates the release of calcium from the bone.

Portions of Food that Give about $\frac{2}{5}$ of USRDA of Calcium

1 cup of whole or skim milk, buttermilk, malted beverage, baked custard, home recipe vanilla or packaged pudding,

yogurt made with partially skim milk, homemade macaroni (enriched) and cheese, potatoes au gratin (with cheese), cooked collards, or 3 ounces of canned sardines

Portions of Food That Give about ⅓ of USRDA of Calcium

1 cup of creamed cottage cheese, soft-serve ice cream or ice milk, cooked cabbage, turnip greens, spoon bread (made with whole ground corn meal), homemade bread pudding, homemade oyster stew, or 1 ounce of Swiss cheese

Portions of Food That Give about ¼ of USRDA of Calcium

1 ounce of process American cheese, 1 cup of uncreamed cottage cheese, hardened ice cream or ice milk, cheese soufflé, lobster Newburg, cooked kale, mustard greens, instant enriched farina (check label), or 1 cup of the following soups made with milk: green pea, cream of celery, cream of mushroom, cream of asparagus

The Calcium Robbers

Rhubarb, spinach, beet greens, and Swiss chard are often called calcium robbers by nutritionists. These foods contain oxalic acid which ties up the calcium so it cannot be used by the body. This is not a serious problem if there is enough calcium in the diet to meet the body's needs. Fortunately, these four foods are not usually eaten in such large quantities that they would cause a serious tie-up of calcium in the body.

Iron

This mineral is often called the mystery mineral. It's a mystery why the body needs such a very small amount of iron to work well, and yet it must have it.

The Handy Food Finder • 75

Iron combines with protein to make hemoglobin and to make myoglobin, which stores oxygen in the muscles for use in muscle movement.

Everyone knows that without enough iron, nutritional anemia develops. Lack of iron also causes metabolic disturbances in the body. Some of the signs of an iron deficiency are a feeling of fatigue, weakness, pale appearance, frequent headaches, and a hemoglobin level lower than normal.

Portions of Food That Give All or More than USRDA of Iron

3 ounces of cooked pork of calf liver, or beef kidney, 1 cup of cooked enriched farina (check labels), 1 cup of prune juice, canned or bottled

Portion of Food That Gives about ⅔ of USRDA of Iron (65 to 70 Percent)

3 ounces cooked beef liver

Portions of Food That Give about ½ of USRDA of Iron (50 to 60 Percent)

4 to 5 raw cherrystone or littleneck clams, 1 cup of (dry) cooked navy beans, lima beans or 1 cup of canned (solid and liquids) white kidney beans, 1 cup of canned pork and sweet sauce baked beans, or 1 cup of drained, canned spinach

Portions of Food That Give about ⅓ of USRDA of Iron

3 ounces of cooked flank steak, lean plate beef, ground lean rump, lean sirloin, lean pork loin, lean beef heart, chicken livers, 1 cup cooked (dry) Great Northern beans, cowpeas or blackeye peas, cooked (dry) whole lentils, cooked (dry) split peas, cooked (dry) soybeans, 1 cup (canned or home recipe) pork and tomato sauce and beans, corned beef hash with potato, chili con carne with beans, home recipe (without noodles) chicken chow mein or beef and pork chop suey,

fresh, frozen or canned lima beans, canned (drained) peas, fresh spinach, home recipe bread pudding with raisins (made with enriched bread), ⅓ of a homemade 9-inch chicken or turkey pot pie (enriched flour) or ⅙ of a 9-inch pecan pie

Portions of Food That Give about ¼ of USRDA of Iron

3 ounces of cooked beef chuck (lean mixed with fat), fresh corned beef, regular or lean ground beef, plate beef (lean and fat), lean rib roast of beef, rump beef, round steak, lean club, porterhouse or T-bone, sirloin (lean and fat), lean cured ham or shoulder cuts (Boston or picnic), fresh ham (lean and fat), fresh pork loin (lean and fat), loin pork chop (lean and fat), fresh shoulder ham, veal as roast or cutlet or ground, canned sardines, boiled shrimp, 1 cup home recipe beef and vegetable stew, or 1 cup of spoon bread made with white whole ground cornmeal, or 1 cup of apple Betty made with enriched bread, or 1 cup of cooked beet greens, Swiss chard, mustard greens, green peas, frozen mixed vegetables (carrots, corn, peas, green beans, snap beans, lima beans), 1 cup of sauerkraut juice, or 10 dried prunes

Foods that contain small amounts of iron that are eaten once a day, or combined with other foods, add up to important amounts of iron in the diet.

For instance, a half-cup of cooked prunes (liquid and fruit) gives about 15 percent of the daily iron needs while 1½ ounces of raisins (about a third of a cup, not pressed down) give about 10 percent of the iron needed daily. You can get about 40 percent of your daily iron in a half-cup of unsweetened, cooked dry apricots, fruit and liquid. Each slice of enriched bread gives about 7 percent of the daily iron needs. An egg provides 10 percent.

It is important to include both the animal and the plant foods that have iron because the body uses the animal sources more efficiently than the plant sources.

Iodine

Lack of iodine in the diet can cause goiter, a swelling of the thyroid gland. However, the regular use of iodized salt as well as sea foods in meals easily provides enough iodine to the body.

Other Minerals

Phosphorus and magnesium play an important role in the development and soundness of teeth and bones. In addition, they are essential in the body's use of food for energy.

Magnesium is found in nuts, whole grains, dark green vegetables, dry beans, and dry peas. When your meals include food rich in protein and calcium, you will get enough phosphorus.

Follow the feel-better plan of eating, based on the Daily Food Guide and the Food Finder, and you will get the ten or more additional minerals important for good health.

A Special Caution

We have described the signs that may show up as a result of shortages of nutrients. But remember, the same signs may also be due to medical disturbances in the body. The body's warnings of disturbances often arise from more than one cause. If, after studying the Food Finder, you make changes in your diet to give you better supplies of certain nutrients, and the signs do not disappear within a relatively short time, then be sure to see your doctor to determine the cause.

Nutrients Often Work Together

We have covered the nutrients one by one for your ready reference, but many nutrients work more often in partnership than individually in the body. This is why the pizza, hamburger, franks and beans diet is so dangerous. There simply aren't enough nutrients to work as partners in doing the body's work for good health.

Here's an example of a dramatic nutrient partnership. Calcium, to be properly absorbed by the body and used to best advantage, must have phosphorus and vitamin D present. It's important to know that all these nutrient partners occur together in vitamin D fortified milk. The after-fifty person who has two glasses (two cups) of milk a day not only gets calcium but receives it along with the partners that can ensure it is used best by the body.

Here's another vital partnership—vitamin C and iron. The body needs a good supply of vitamin C to help it absorb and make the best use of iron. Vitamin C helps change the iron to a form in which the body can use it easily. When the "C" is not present, less of the iron is put to work in the body.

Vitamin E works with other substances in the body to protect both vitamin A and carotene from being destroyed.

There are many other nutrient partnerships too complicated to include here. These are just a few examples that point up the tremendous importance of having a wide variety of foods in the day's meals. Besides, it's so much more exciting than eating the same old thing!

We suggest that you study this Food Finder carefully. It will give you much information about food for feeling better. Notice which foods are richest in nutrients. Pick out your favorites and write them down to remind you to serve them often. It's the feel-better way.

8
A Simple Eating Guide

Now that we know the nitty-gritty of nutrients, it's time to turn to a very simple plan for good eating, the Daily Food Guide of the United States Department of Agriculture. It's divided into four basic food groups. When you boil down the complicated science of nutrition to only four food groups, there are some drawbacks. The guide can't cover everything, but it is an excellent way to check what foods a person needs daily. Here's the guide:

A Daily Food Guide*

Meat Group

Foods Included. Beef, veal, lamb, pork, variety meats (such as liver, heart, kidney), poultry and eggs, fish and shellfish. *As alternates*—dry beans, dry peas, lentils, nuts, peanuts, peanut butter.

Amounts Recommended. Choose 2 or more servings every day. Count as a serving: 2 to 3 ounces of lean cooked meat, poultry, or fish—all without bone. One egg; ½ cup cooked dry beans, dry peas, or lentils; 2 tablespoons of peanut butter may replace one-half serving of meat.

* From U.S. Department of Agriculture Home and Garden Bulletin #1.

Vegetable-Fruit Group

Foods Included. All vegetables and fruits. This guide emphasizes those that are valuable as sources of vitamin C and vitamin A.

Sources of Vitamin C. Good sources—Grapefruit or grapefruit juice, orange or orange juice, cantaloupe, guava, mango, papaya, raw strawberries, broccoli, brussels sprouts, green pepper, sweet red pepper.

Fair Sources—Honeydew melon, lemon, tangerine or tangerine juice, watermelon, asparagus, cabbage, collards, garden cress, kale, kohlrabi, mustard greens, potatoes and sweet potatoes cooked in the jacket, spinach, tomatoes or tomato juice, turnip greens.

Sources of Vitamin A. Dark-green and deep-yellow vegetables and a few fruits—namely, apricots, broccoli, cantaloupe, carrots, chard, collards, cress, kale, mango, persimmon, pumpkin, spinach, sweet potatoes, turnip greens and other dark-green leaves, winter squash.

Amounts Recommended. Choose 4 or more servings every day, including 1 serving of a good source of vitamin C or 2 servings of a fair source and 1 serving, at least every other day, of a good source of vitamin A (if the food chosen for vitamin C is also a good source of vitamin A, the additional serving of a vitamin A food may be omitted). The remaining 1 to 3 or more servings may be of any vegetable or fruit, including those that are valuable for vitamin C and for vitamin A. Count as 1 serving: ½ cup of vegetable or fruit, or a portion as ordinarily served, such as 1 medium apple, banana, orange, or potato, half a medium grapefruit or cantaloupe, or the juice of 1 lemon.

Milk Group

Foods Included. Milk (fluid whole, evaporated, skim, dry, buttermilk), cheese (cottage, cream, Cheddar-type, natural or process), ice cream.

A Simple Eating Guide • 81

Amounts Recommended. Some milk every day for everyone. Recommended amounts are given below in terms of 8-ounce cups of whole fluid milk:

Children under 9 (2 to 3)   Adults (2 or more)
Children 9 to 12 (3 or more)   Pregnant women (3 or more)
Teen-agers (4 or more)   Nursing mothers (4 or more)

Part or all of the milk may be fluid skim milk, buttermilk, evaporated milk, or dry milk. Cheese and ice cream may replace part of the milk. The amount of either it will take to replace a given amount of milk is figured on the basis of calcium content. Common portions of cheese and of ice cream and their milk equivalents in calcium are:

1-inch cube Cheddar-type cheese	½ cup of milk
½ cup of cottage cheese	⅓ cup of milk
2 tablespoons of cream cheese	1 tablespoon of milk
½ cup of ice cream or ice milk	⅓ cup of milk

Bread-Cereal Group

Foods Included. All breads and cereals that are whole grain, enriched, or restored; *check labels to be sure.* Specifically, this group includes breads, cooked cereals, ready-to-eat cereals, cornmeal, crackers, flour, grits, macaroni and spaghetti, noodles, rice, rolled oats, and quick breads and other baked goods if made with whole grain or enriched flour. Bulgur and parboiled rice and wheat also may be included in this group.

Amounts Recommended. Choose 4 servings or more daily. Or, if no cereals are chosen, have an extra serving of breads or baked goods, which will make at least 5 servings from this group daily. Count as 1 serving: 1 slice of bread; 1 ounce of ready-to-eat cereal; ½ to ¾ cup of cooked cereal, cornmeal, grits, macaroni, noodles, rice, or spaghetti.

Other Foods

To round out meals and meet energy needs, almost everyone will use some foods not specified in the four food groups.

Such foods include: unenriched, refined breads, cereals, flours, sugars, butter, margarine, other fats. These often are ingredients in a recipe or added to other foods during preparation or at the table. Try to include some vegetable oil among the fats used.

One drawback to this guide is that except in the Vegetable-Fruit Group, the main nutrients in the foods, and the amounts in which they are found, are not given. We also feel that in this group, where four or more servings are recommended, at least two of the servings should be vegetables.

Here's another problem. As seen in the Food Finder, the amount of nutrients in different foods may swing all the way from providing the entire day's need for a nutrient to only a fourth. This guide doesn't show such differences, but you can easily check them out in the Food Finder, and make your choices from the basic four food groups accordingly.

Then, too, this guide cannot cover special foods such as those eaten by cultural, social, and religious groups who follow ethnic traditions or religious restrictions in their diets. These foods are too numerous to include in a simple basic guide. Some would be hard to fit into any one food group. Here again, the Food Finder will be helpful for opening up more food sources of important nutrients to fit every person's persuasion and taste.

As you will note, this guide is built mostly around individual foods as they come from nature: fruits, vegetables, meats, milk, cheese, bread, and cereals. But today we live in a different world. Many foods at the supermarket are combined in products such as TV dinners, prepackaged main dishes, rice mixes, add-your-own-meat mixes, etc. These products are impossible to include by nutrient content in any one basic food group. They may straddle all four and still fit nowhere. This confuses people trying to choose foods that give the nutrients they need in their meals.

A Simple Eating Guide • 83

Main Nutrients in the Basic Four Food Groups

Since the guide does not give the main nutrients in all four food groups, here is a quick review.

The milk group is a primary source of calcium and also provides riboflavin, protein, phosphorus, as well as vitamin D when milk is fortified. Check milk container labels.

The meat group (which should really be called the protein group) gives proteins, iron, phosphorus, and the B vitamins: thiamine, riboflavin, and niacin.

The vegetable and fruit group is a primary source of vitamin C, and also provides vitamin A, some iron, and other minerals. This group also gives fiber (cellulose or roughage) important for efficient elimination.

The bread-cereal group provides many of the B vitamins, iron, carbohydrates, and cellulose.

Notice how the nutrients overlap in the four food groups. There is iron in the protein group; some iron is available in the fruit and vegetable group; and also in the bread and cereal group. As we saw in "The Handy Food Finder," chapter 7, only a few foods, such as calf and pork liver, provide all of the iron needed daily. Iron has to be gotten in small amounts from several foods in a day's meals. Getting the day's nutrients in a variety of foods also puts much less strain on the pocketbook.

The Menu Game

When the Feel-Better Group was first finding its way through a lot of food information that was new, we found it helpful to play a simple game to get our bearings. The name of the game was "What's Missing from This Menu?"

Here's a menu:

Tuna Sandwich
Glass of Milk

What's missing?

There's no food from the fruit and vegetable group. Since you need four or more servings a day from this group, it's almost impossible to get them if you leave a fruit or vegetable out of one meal. Add to this menu a piece of fresh fruit and some raw vegetable sticks. That does it.

Here's another menu:

    Peanut Butter Sandwich
    Carrot Sticks
    Orange
    Oatmeal Cookie
    Tea

What's missing?

There's nothing from the milk group. A cup of milk is particularly needed in this menu to improve the quality of the incomplete protein in the peanut butter as well as to provide calcium and riboflavin.

Another menu:

    Cottage Cheese Fruit Salad
    Tea

There's nothing here from the bread and cereal group to give additional bulk, as well as B vitamins and some iron. You may have responded, as did some members of the Feel-Better Group, that there is nothing from the meat group in this menu. True. But you get about 20 percent of your complete protein needs for the day in a tightly packed quarter-cup of cottage cheese (pressed down). Many of the foods in the milk group are very good sources of complete protein and can be used to supply the same protein as is found in meat, but you would never know it from the Daily Food Guide. There, cheese is presented in the milk group. It is not stated that cheese, such as American or Cheddar, is interchangeable with meat for complete protein. Again, you would never know from this guide that macaroni and cheese made with milk will make just as good a main dish for dinner as a hamburger patty, and it may be cheaper. To add to the confusion, the macaroni is found in the bread and cereals group of the daily guide, yet it is a source of incomplete protein. This is an important nutrient when improved by the addition of milk or cheese, or both, as in macaroni and cheese in a home recipe.

The Daily Food Guide is a good way to check that you are getting the right foods and enough of them, but use it in combination with the Handy Food Finder to get the best results in planning feel-better meals.

9
Fourteen Days of Feel-Better Food: Passkeys to Livelier Living

HERE ARE TWO WEEKS of feel-better meals, planned to bring all the foods needed in just the right combinations to do the most good for your body.

These are not just menus. They are a way of life. They combine the best of the science and wisdom of good eating as it is understood today.

The world where we human beings live adds up in a wonderful way. Inside our bodies are the working parts for a life, a marvelous machine that works well when treated right. Outside of us is the earth, and the earth gives all that we need for life: fruits . . . vegetables . . . meats . . . grains . . . with their vitamins, minerals, protein, carbohydrates, and fats. To fulfill the bond between our bodies and the earth, we must eat the good foods that the earth offers. That's when our bodies work well and we feel well. It's called good health. It's living on earth as we were meant to do for our own good.

When you hold a round orange or an apple in your hand, you hold a sun and a moon of life itself. When you look down at your dinner plate—the meat, the vegetable, the potato, the salad, the bread, and milk to drink with it— it is your present and your future set out before you; you can feel no better than the food that you eat. If you look down on your plate and you see junk food, that's how you'll feel—junky.

It's a fact that 400 million people in the world go to bed hungry every night. We are lucky to live in a land of abundance. Use the fruits of our ample farms and ranges wisely to keep well and to renew the body. Good eating will lift the spirits, too. It is one of the greatest gifts during our time on earth, especially to be treasured in the later years.

Here are the menus that put it all together in a way to do most good. Menus, and recipes to match (pages 190-206) are planned to serve one person since so many after-fifty people live alone.

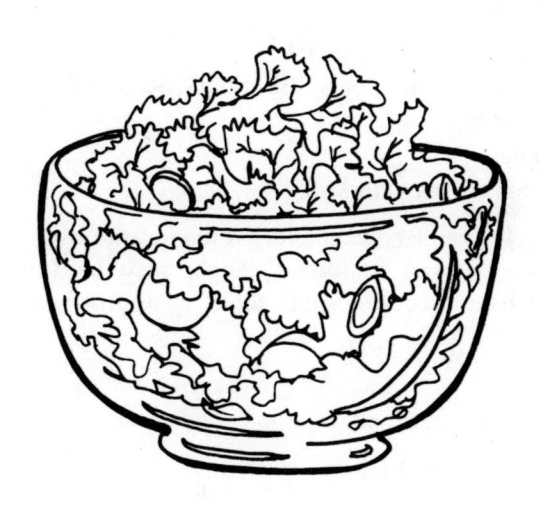

Breakfast

Sliced Peaches
Whole Wheat Flakes with Milk
Whole Wheat Bread and Spread
Coffee or Tea with Milk

Variations
Choice of Spread. Butter, margarine, or cottage cheese.

Main Dish Variation. In place of whole wheat flakes with milk, use ¼ cup of cottage cheese or ¾ cup of yogurt mixed with peach slices.

Milk: Drink ½ cup separately if not used in coffee or tea.

Peaches. Fresh or canned.

Lunch

Chopped Liver Sandwich
Raw Vegetables (page 131) Sticks, Strips, Circles, or Grated
Apple
Coffee or Tea with Milk

Note. Liver sandwich filling is made from liver that comes with chicken served at dinner. Apple may be fresh, or unsweetened baked, cooked apple slices, or applesauce.

Dinner

Chicken with Rice
Broccoli
Mixed Vegetable Salad
Bread
Pudding Topped with Fruit
Coffee or Tea with Milk

Work Savers. Serving fresh fruit saves work. Cook chicken and rice in one pot to save dishwashing and fuel.

Fourteen Days of Feel-Better Food • 89

Breakfast

Orange Juice
Farina or Cream of Wheat with Milk
Whole Wheat Bread with Spread
Coffee or Tea with Milk

Variation. Peanut butter sandwich instead of farina and bread. Increase milk to 1 cup.

Lunch

Salad Plate of Cottage Cheese, Peach Slices and No-Cook Prunes on Greens
Banana Bread
Coffee or Tea with Milk

Variation. Use yogurt or ricotta cheese in place of cottage cheese.

Dinner

Meat Loaf
Potatoes Boiled in Skin
Spinach or other Vitamin A-rich vegetable
Vegetable Salad
Bread
Pear
Coffee or Tea with Milk

Work Savers. Cooking potatoes unpeeled means more nutrition, more flavor, and saves work and waste. Buying small potatoes cuts down cooking time, saves money on utility bills.

The meat loaf is both a time saver and a super work saver. The same meat loaf recipe makes three or four meals. It's served sliced at one dinner; cold in a sandwich at another; and in spaghetti and meat balls at still another meal. The meat loaf mixture in this case is baked partly as a meat loaf, and partly as meatballs in the same pan.

Make Banana Bread when you feel like baking; cut into slices, wrap, and freeze for future use. One loaf makes 12 to 16 slices.

Breakfast

No-Cook Prunes
Egg
Whole Wheat Bread and Spread
Coffee or Tea with Milk

Lunch

Meat Loaf Sandwich
Broccoli Salad
Pudding
   Topped with Peaches
Coffee or Tea with Milk

Dinner

Top-of-Stove Macaroni and Cheese
Stewed Tomatoes
Mixed Vegetable Salad
Bread
Fruit Cup
Coffee or Tea with Milk

Work Savers. Broccoli Salad: when cooking vegetables, make a little extra to be used in salads within a couple of days.

Macaroni and Cheese is made in a saucepan on top of the stove instead of in the oven, to save time, fuel, and messy dishwashing.

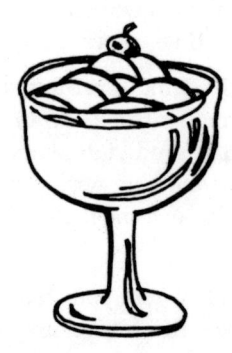

Breakfast

Grapefruit Half
Whole Wheat Flakes with Milk
Whole Wheat Bread with Spread
Coffee or Tea with Milk

Variation. Milk toast in place of cereal and bread.

Lunch

Bean Soup
Spinach and Egg-Fry
Bread
Piece of Fresh Fruit
Coffee or Tea with Milk

Dinner

Pan-Fried Fish
Mixed Vegetables or Peas
Tossed Green Salad
Top-of-Stove Bread Pudding
Coffee or Tea with Milk

Work Saver. Make Bread Pudding in advance.

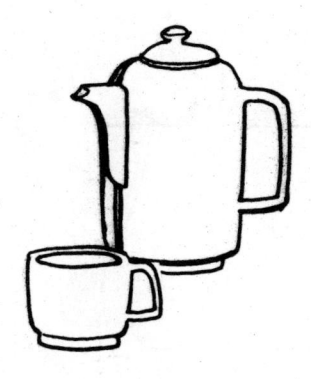

Breakfast

Feel-Better Breakfast in a Drink (page 30)
Whole Wheat Bread with Spread
Coffee or Tea, if desired

Variation. Use a bran muffin in place of the bread. Make a batch; freeze the extras for future use.

Lunch

Cottage Cheese Combo Sandwich
Raw Spinach Salad
Piece of Fresh Fruit
Coffee or Tea with Milk

Dinner

Spaghetti and Meatballs
Broccoli or other Vitamin A-rich vegetable
Raw Vegetable Sticks
Grapefruit Half
Coffee or Tea with Milk

Work Saver. Spaghetti and Meatballs are made with Meat Loaf recipe on page 192.

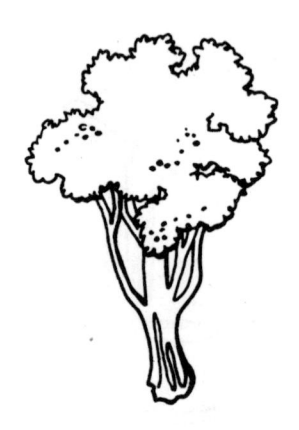

Breakfast

Prune Juice
Bread Pudding with Milk
Coffee or Tea with Milk

Note. Serve Pudding either heated or cold.

Lunch

Put-Together "Stoup" or Lima Bean-Cheese Quickie
Mixed Green Salad
Bread
Coffee or Tea with Milk

Note. "Stoup" is neither stew nor soup but a combination of leftovers from other meals, eaten in a soup bowl.

Dinner

Roast Chicken
Summer or Winter Squash
Oven Roasted Potatoes
Tomato Salad
Bread
Fresh Fruit
Coffee or Tea with Milk

Work Saver. Cook extra chicken to make chicken salad for another meal. Save chicken drippings for future use.

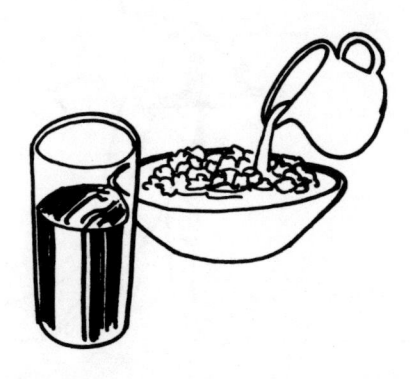

Breakfast
Orange Juice
Scrambled Egg
Toast with Spread
Coffee or Tea with Milk

Note. Egg may be boiled or eaten in a sandwich.

Lunch
Bean Soup
Chicken Salad on Greens
Bread
Fruit Cup
Coffee or Tea with Milk

Dinner
Cook's Choice
Protein food of your choice such as meat, cheese, fish, chicken (pages 44-47)
Vitamin A-rich Vegetable (pages 59-60)
Rice, Noodles or Potatoes
Salad
Bread
Dessert of your choice
Coffee or Tea with Milk

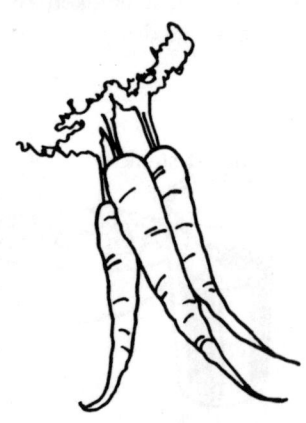

Breakfast

Prune Juice
Ready-to-Eat Cereal with Milk
Whole Wheat Bread with Spread
Coffee or Tea with Milk

Variation. Instead of cereal and bread, use a cold meat or fish sandwich made from leftovers.

Lunch

Peanut Butter-Cottage Cheese Sandwich
Raw Vegetables
Orange
Cup of Milk
Coffee or Tea

Dinner

Pan Broiled Steak
Potato Boiled in Skin
Carrots
Mixed Green Salad
Bread
Apple
Coffee or Tea with Milk

Note. You can afford steak when you use the beef cutting plan (pages 151-153) in which beef chuck blade steak is divided at home for small beef cuts at much less money. In these menus, the steak dinner, the steak sandwich, and the beef stir-fry are all made from one beef chuck blade steak cut up at home. Save pan drippings.

Work Saver. When cooking steak, cook a small extra portion for a steak sandwich at another meal. Refrigerate until ready to use.

Breakfast

Tomato Juice
Farina, Oatmeal, or Cream of Wheat with Milk
Whole Wheat Bread with Spread
Coffee or Tea with Milk

Lunch

Vegetable Beef Soup
Egg Salad on Greens
Bread Pudding
Coffee or Tea with Milk

Dinner

Broiled Chicken
Potato
Broccoli or other Vitamin A-rich Vegetable
Mixed-Lima and Kidney Bean Salad
Bread
Stewed Fruit
Coffee or Tea with Milk

Work Savers. Broil half a chicken; eat one serving for dinner. Refrigerate the two remaining servings, or freeze them. Use to make chicken sandwich for lunch, and a creamed chicken dinner dish. Saves time, energy, and cuts down on fuel bills.

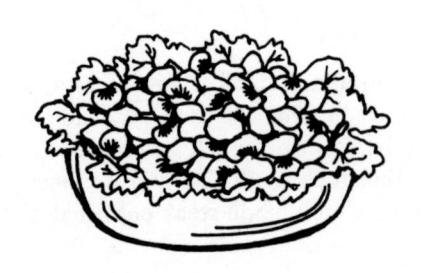

Breakfast

Grapefruit Half
Ready-to-Eat Cereal such as Bran Cereal with Milk
Whole Wheat Bread with Spread
Coffee or Tea with ½ Cup Milk

Variation. Mix cereal with yogurt instead of milk.

Lunch

Steak Sandwich
Broccoli Salad
Peach Slices
Coffee or Tea with Milk

Dinner

Homemade Pizza
Big Mixed Green and Cooked Vegetable Salad
Fruit Cup
Cup of Milk
Coffee or Tea

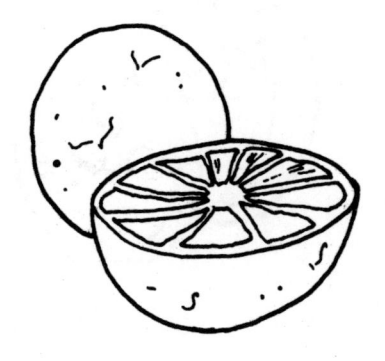

Breakfast

Feel-Better Breakfast in a Drink (page 30)
Whole Wheat Bread with Spread
Coffee or Tea, if desired

Lunch

Chicken Sandwich
Fresh Spinach Salad
Apple or Plums
Coffee or Tea with Milk

Dinner

Stir-Fry Beef on Rice
Green Beans or Mixed Vegetables
Tossed Green Salad
Bread
Ice Cream or
Stewed Fruit
Coffee or Tea with Milk

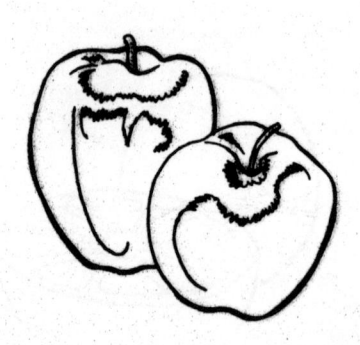

Breakfast

Tomato Juice
Egg
Whole Wheat Bread with Spread
Coffee or Tea with ½ Cup of Milk

Lunch

Liver Spread Sandwich
Raw Vegetables
Plums or other Fresh Fruit
Coffee or Tea with Milk

Dinner

Old-Fashioned Fish Chowder
Carrot/Cabbage Slaw
Bread
Fruit Cup and Oatmeal Cookies
Coffee or Tea with Milk

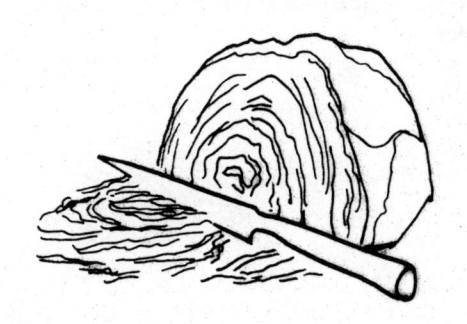

Breakfast

Orange Juice
Farina with Milk
Banana Bread
Coffee or Tea with Milk

Lunch

Bean Soup
Cottage Cheese and Vegie Combo Sandwich
Green Bean Salad
Fresh Fruit
Coffee or Tea with Milk

Dinner

Creamed Chicken
Noodles
Spinach or other Vitamin A-rich Vegetable
Mixed Vegetable Salad
Bread
Peach or Apricots
Coffee or Tea with Milk

Note. White sauce recipe for creamed chicken on page 196.

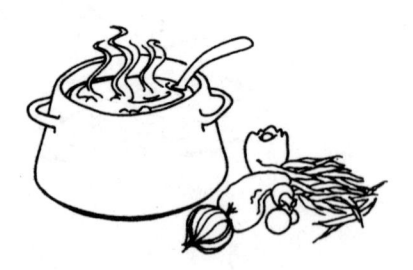

Breakfast

No-Cook Prunes
Oatmeal with Milk
Whole Wheat Bread with Spread
Coffee or Tea with Milk

Lunch

Vegetable Soup
Tuna Sandwich
Raw Vegetables
Orange
Coffee or Tea with Milk

Dinner

Cook's Choice
Protein Food of your choice such as meat, cheese, fish, chicken
Vitamin A-rich Vegetable (pages 59-60)
Rice, Noodles or Potatoes
Salad
Bread
Dessert of your choice
Coffee or Tea with Milk

10
Never Have to Diet Again

HERE'S A SHOCKER. In a ten-state nutrition survey made by the U.S. Government, it was found that 50 percent of the older women surveyed were dangerously overweight. Here's another shocker. Men 45 years of age of medium height and frame, weighing 170 pounds, have a life expectancy of 1½ years less than men of comparable build who weigh 150 pounds, which is within the desirable range of weights. Those weighing 200 pounds, or 35 pounds above the average, can expect to live 4 years less. Thus we see that by carrying 20 pounds less weight, a person in normal health can live considerably longer!

One never reads a death notice in the newspaper that says a man died of overweight, but it is true that overweight is dangerous to a person's health, especially when he or she is suffering from heart disease, hypertension, diabetes, or other serious diseases.

How Much Weight Is Overweight?

Some people think that it's just natural to be fat when you're over fifty. Not so, or at least not in most cases. There are certain diseases such as active tuberculosis, or chronic ulcerative colitis where a mild degree of overweight is desirable. In some cases, the psychological effects of reducing are more damaging to the person than the overweight itself. This is why it is a "must" to see a doctor before taking on any reducing plan. Once it was thought that if a person weighed 10 percent to 19 percent more than the average for his height and body build, he was overweight. If he weighed 20 percent or more above the average, he was considered obese. Nutritionists now consider that if 30 percent or less of his body weight is in fat cells, a person is considered normal; if 40 percent or more is in fat cells, he is considered obese. If in between, the person is considered overweight. Ten pounds or more over standard weight should be taken off by the person. The higher go the pounds over the ideal weight, the harder it is to get rid of them. Most people, including the authors, know that from experience.

A look in the mirror, without clothes, will tell most people when they are overweight. If you've done that, and don't like what you see, double-check overweight by giving yourself the pinch test or the ruler test.

For the pinch test, stand up and pinch the flesh right under the ribs in front. If the thickness of flesh between the fingers is less than one inch, you probably aren't fat. If it is more than an inch, it's a sign that it's time to reduce.

Or try the ruler test. Lie down without clothes and put a ruler on your body from your chest to your tummy. If the ruler lies perfectly flat and there is a little space underneath where you can put your hand in between the ends of the ruler, you're not overweight. But if the ruler lies on a slant uphill or downhill, it's time to think about losing a few pounds.

How Many Calories?

Constant calorie counting is unnecessary for those who eat wisely. But you may wish to know the general rule for the desirable number of daily calories for a man or a woman

DESIRABLE WEIGHTS—AGES 25 AND OVER*
Weight in Pounds According to Frame (In Indoor Clothing)

Men

Height (with shoes on) 1-inch heels Feet Inches	Small Frame	Medium Frame	Large Frame
5 2	112–120	118–129	126–141
5 3	115–123	121–133	129–144
5 4	118–126	124–136	132–148
5 5	121–129	127–139	135–152
5 6	124–133	130–143	138–156
5 7	128–137	134–147	142–161
5 8	132–141	138–152	147–166
5 9	136–145	142–156	151–170
5 10	140–150	146–160	155–174
5 11	144–154	150–165	159–179
6 0	148–158	154–170	164–184
6 1	152–162	158–175	168–189
6 2	156–167	162–180	173–194
6 3	160–171	167–185	178–199
6 4	164–175	172–190	182–204

*Chart courtesy of Metropolitan Life Insurance Company.

Women

Height (with shoes on) 2-inch heels Feet Inches	Small Frame	Medium Frame	Large Frame
4 10	92– 98	96–107	104–119
4 11	94–101	98–110	106–122
5 0	96–104	101–113	109–125
5 1	99–107	104–116	112–128
5 2	102–110	107–119	115–131
5 3	105–113	110–122	118–134
5 4	108–116	113–126	121–138
5 5	111–119	116–130	125–142
5 6	114–123	120–135	129–146
5 7	118–127	124–139	133–150
5 8	122–131	128–143	137–154
5 9	126–135	132–147	141–158
5 10	130–140	136–151	145–163
5 11	134–144	140–155	149–168
6 0	138–148	144–159	153–173

For girls between 18 and 25, subtract 1 pound for each year under 25.

over fifty. As mentioned, metabolism slows down after fifty, so calories must be reduced, too, to keep the weight right.

The U.S. Recommended Daily Allowances for calories for a man fifty and over are 2,400, and 1,800 for a woman. There may be slight differences in calorie needs, depending upon body composition and size, age, and activity of the person.

Why Most Diets Don't Work

Most reducing diets will take off pounds, but they don't stay off. That's because people haven't changed their food habits for the better. Until they do, the weight comes right back. Then, too, some freaky diets can have dangerous side effects, especially for older people. If diets cause a person to lose more than one or two pounds a week, they may make him or her feel weak, and put a serious strain on the body. Large weight losses in a short period of time may result in the skin becoming more wrinkled, particularly in older people. Fad diets and fast weight losses can also result in depression, irritability, and in being generally hard to live with. Besides, people normally get too hungry on these diets and go on food binges that bring back the weight lost, and put on extra pounds.

The Amazing News

Overweight people in normal health who shift to the feel-better meals given in the previous chapter *will lose about three-quarters of a pound a week!* That's because they change their food habits. They are giving the body just what it needs in the right amounts to do its work. By the way, the *amounts* are just as important as the kinds of food eaten, so follow the directions given in chapter 6 and in the Daily Food Guide, chapter 8, for the right amount of food for people after fifty.

With feel-better meals, you won't be tempted to go off your diet because the meals are varied, appetizing, satisfying.

And they are planned to keep the body spinning along at its right weight.

For those in normal health who are not seriously overweight, regular feel-better menus will do the trick. For others, the doctor must be consulted to work out a regime to get the pounds off. Then they can go on feel-better meals, and keep the weight off, if the doctor agrees.

For those few who do not lose about a pound a week on regular feel-better meals, make these changes:

1. Use skim milk instead of whole milk.

2. Reduce the amount of fat to just 3 small servings. A serving of fat is 1½ teaspoons of butter, margarine, vegetable oil, or other clear fat; or 1 level tablespoon light cream, half and half, or sour cream; or 1 level tablespoon of French or Italian salad dressing.

3. Use broiled, baked, or boiled lean protein foods such as meat, chicken, fish. Limit the amount to 4 or 5 ounces. The following may be used as alternates for 1 ounce of cooked protein foods: about ¼ cup tuna, 1 ounce of salmon, 1 ounce of crabmeat or lobster, 1 egg, ¼ cup of cottage cheese, about 4 medium size oysters, 4 medium shrimp, 4 medium clams, 1 cup of skim milk, 1 8-ounce container of yogurt.

4. In place of ice cream and puddings in the regular feel-better menus, use unsweetened fruits.

You will notice that we use no special diet foods in our menus. You may have tried such so-called diet products as frozen main dishes prepared with very little fat, or fruits canned with sugar substitute. Low-fat dishes can be made at home at much less expense. Cooking in a small amount of fat is the healthful thing to do all year around, not just on a reducing diet. Fruits are delicious eaten without sugar. People who base their temporary reducing diets on special diet foods usually gain back all the weight when they drop

REDUCING GUIDE FOR PEOPLE IN NORMAL HEALTH TO LOSE 1 TO 2 POUNDS A WEEK

DAILY MENU PATTERN

SAMPLE MENUS

Breakfast

Fruit, unsweetened	
Egg and bread, or cereal with ½ cup of skim milk	
Coffee or tea with ½ cup of skim milk	

Lunch

Protein food
Vegetable
Bread
Fruit
Milk, skim

Dinner

Protein food
Vegetables, 2 or more servings, 1 cooked, 1 or more raw
Salad dressing
Bread, 1 slice
Fruit, 1 piece
Coffee or tea with ½ cup of skim milk

Breakfast

Orange juice, unsweetened	½ cup
Farina with skim milk	½ cup
Coffee or tea with skim milk	½ cup

Lunch

Sandwich	
American cheese	1 ounce
Whole wheat bread	1 slice
Carrot sticks	1 carrot
Peach, fresh or canned, unsweetened	1
Milk, skim	1 cup

Dinner

Broiled hamburger	3 oz. cooked
Broccoli	½ cup
Mixed green salad	2 to 3 servings
Salad dressing	1½ teaspoons
Whole wheat bread	1 slice
Apple	1 medium
Coffee or tea with ½ cup of skim milk	½ cup

Breakfast

Grapefruit	½ small
Hard or soft boiled egg	1
Whole wheat toast	1 slice
Butter or margarine	1 level teaspoon
Coffee or tea with skim milk	½ cup

Lunch

Salad	
Cottage cheese	⅓ cup
Tomato	1
Salad greens	1 to 2 servings
Dressing	1 teaspoon
Whole wheat bread	1 slice
Prunes, unsweetened	3
Milk, skim	1 cup

Dinner

Broiled chicken	Leg or breast
Spinach	½ cup
Mixed green salad	2 to 3 servings
Dressing	1½ teaspoons
Bread	1 slice
Cantaloupe	¼ medium
Coffee or tea with skim milk	½ cup

Tips for zestier taste. Add to raw salads or cooked vegetables, fresh parsley, basil, chives, green or red pepper, fennel, dill, lemon or onion juice, or tomato juice. Make salad dressings using buttermilk, or yogurt as base. Flavor with pickle, lemon or tomato juice, dry mustard or paprika, garlic. Limit oil, if added, to 1½ to 2 teaspoons.

their special diet foods, and return to eating the foods that put the weight on in the first place.

Keeping It Off

When you have gotten down to your best weight (Oh, happy day!), and are still losing each week, continue eating the feel-better way, but increase the amounts of food a little until you are eating just enough to keep your weight steady. For example, if you reach 135 pounds and that's where you should stay, add a half-cup of pudding to one meal and some peas at another meal during a week. If you still continue to lose weight, add a cup of your favorite soup to a meal, and a half-cup of green beans to another meal during the week. Once you reach the point where your weight is correct, and where you are not losing or gaining, you know this is the right amount of food for you for feeling better.

Two Basic Reducing Patterns

Here are a daily meal pattern and sample menus for two days to help reduce while eating nutritious foods. These are the safe amounts to eat daily. You may have noticed that we do not use bouillon in our menus. There is a reason why. It is high in salt, and salt often causes problems for older people. It is linked with water retention in the body (edema), and with hypertension, and other undesirable conditions. It is better to make your own beef or chicken broth with very little salt and rely for flavoring on added vegetables such as carrots, onion, celery, peas. Be sure to skim off the fat before using the broth.

Tips to Help You Get Your Weight Down

Once you've seen your doctor and worked out a reducing plan, these tips may help:

1. Set realistic goals for yourself. Concentrate on losing the first five pounds. When you reach that goal, then go after the next five pounds, and so on.

2. Weigh youself just once a week on the same scale wearing about the same weight of clothing. Keep a written record of the date, your weight, and the time of day you weighed. It is best to weigh yourself before breakfast. Some people find it good to write down everything eaten each day. It helps them to stay on their diet. Few people realize all the extras they eat—the very items that are putting on the pounds.

3. If you aren't already an active person, it's important to increase your activity. Choose some form of activity you enjoy, and gradually increase the amount of time in which you do it. For example, if you drive to the stores, park at the farthest end of the parking lot and walk from there. The idea is to keep moving! If you sweep off the porch twice a week, give it a going-over four or five times a week. If you like to dance and haven't done so in years, invite a friend to your home, and dance for ten or twenty minutes at a time. Better still, if you belong to a community center, ask that the record player be put on for twenty to twenty-five minutes after mealtime, and encourage people to dance. For those who ride a bicycle, increase the amount by riding another five minutes. Some people find exercises helpful. However, the same thing can be accomplished by walking, bending while doing work such as housework, or becoming involved in activities that take people outside the home. A diet of sitting for long hours in front of the TV screen, or playing cards or bingo, is neither a reducing diet nor a feel-better diet.

A Road Map of Calorie Land

Just to help you steer clear of foods heavy in calories, here is a listing of basic foods and the calories they contain. The same foods often come in a form with fewer calories, and may be better for you. For instance, skim milk has only

90 calories in a cup while whole milk has 150 calories. Both are fine foods. In some cases, to keep weight down, it may be better to drink the skim milk, which does not have the fat. Again, three ounces of chicken broiled without the skin have only 120 calories while three ounces of lean beef rib roast have 210 calories. Enjoy both in your meals. Be sure to include the chicken, which has fewer calories, as well as the roast beef, or other beef that you like.

A calorie, as you know, is simply a measure of the amount of energy, or heat, given off by a food when it burns in the body. When there are more calories in meals than the body needs, the extra calories are stored as fat.

Check, too, to see that calories are keeping company with a good amount of vitamins, minerals, and protein so that the calories will bring important nutrition to the body. Foods such as candies, most cakes, and soft drinks add calories with little or no nutrition. They tend to crowd out other important foods that are needed by the body. They satisfy hunger or thirst without giving the body the nutrients it needs to work properly.

THE CALORIE LAND ROAD MAP
(TO HELP YOU WATCH OUT FOR EXTRA CURVES!)

Dairy Products	Amount	Calories
Cheese		
Cheddar	1 ounce	115
Cottage, creamed	1 ounce	30
Mozzarella	1 ounce	90
Parmesan, grated	1 tablespoon	25
American, pasteurized process	1 ounce	105
Swiss	1 ounce	105
Cream		
Half and Half	1 tablespoon	20
Light, coffee or table	1 tablespoon	30
Heavy whipping, unwhipped	1 tablespoon	80
Light whipping, unwhipped	1 tablespoon	45
Sour cream	1 tablespoon	25

Dairy (cont.)	Amount	Calories
Milk		
Fluid		
Whole	1 cup	150
Low fat (2%)	1 cup	120
Skim	1 cup	90
Buttermilk	1 cup	100
Milk drinks		
Chocolate, regular	1 cup	210
Eggnog	1 cup	340
Malted	1 cup	235
Milk desserts		
Ice cream		
Regular	1/2 cup	135
Soft serve	1/2 cup	185
Ice milk		
Hardened	1/2 cup	90
Soft serve	1/2 cup	110
Custard, baked	1/2 cup	150
Vanilla pudding (blanc mange)	1/2 cup	145
Regular chocolate pudding (mix)		
Cooked	1/2 cup	160
Instant	1/2 cup	165
Yogurt made with low fat milk		
Fruit flavored	8-ounce carton	230
Plain	8-ounce carton	145

Eggs

Large	1 egg	80
Egg white	1 white	15
Egg yolk	1 yolk	65
Fried in butter	1 egg	85
Poached	1 egg	80
Scrambled, with milk and butter	1 egg	95

Fats, Oils, and Related Products

Butter	1 tablespoon	100
Lard	1 tablespoon	115
Margarine	1 tablespoon	100
Vegetable oils	1 tablespoon	120
French dressing, commercial	1 tablespoon	65
Italian dressing, commercial	1 tablespoon	85
Mayonnaise, commercial	1 tablespoon	100

Fish and Shellfish	Amount	Calories
Bluefish, baked with butter	3 ounces	135
Clams		
Raw	3 ounces	65
Canned (solids and liquid)	3 ounces	45
Crabmeat	1/2 cup	65
Fish sticks, frozen, cooked	1-ounce stick	50
Haddock, breaded, fried	3 ounces	140
Shrimp, canned	3 ounces	100
Tuna, canned in oil, drained	3 ounces	170

Meats

	Amount	Calories
Ground beef, cooked		
Lean, with 10% fat	3 ounces	185
Lean, with 21% fat	2.9 ounces	235
Beef rib roast		
Fat and lean	3 ounces	375
Lean only	3 ounces	125
Corned beef, canned	3 ounces	185
Corned beef, hash, canned	1 cup	400
Beef and vegetable stew, canned	1 cup	220
Beef pot pie, homemade		
(9-inch diameter)	1/3 of pie	515
Chili con carne with beans	1 cup	340
Lamb leg		
Roasted, lean and fat	3 ounces	235
Lean only	3 ounces	130
Pork, roasted		
Lean and fat	3 ounces	310
Lean only	3 ounces	175
Bologna, 1 slice	1 ounce	85
Deviled ham, canned, (slightly less than ½ ounce)	1 level tablespoon	45
Frankfurter (2 ounces each)	1 frankfurter	170
Chicken		
Broiled, boned	6.2 ounces	240
Breast, fried, boned	2.8 ounces	160
Drumstick, fried, boned	1.3 ounces	90
Canned boneless	3 ounces	170
Chicken a la king, homemade	1 cup	470
Chicken and noodled, homemade	1 cup	365
Chicken pot pie, homemade (9-inch diameter, about 3 cups)	1/3 of pie	545
Turkey, cooked	3 ounces	160
chopped or diced	1 cup	265

Fruit and Fruit Products	Amount	Calories
Apple, raw (3 per pound, 2¾ inches in diameter)	1 apple	80
Apple juice	1 cup	120
Applesauce		
Sweetened	1/2 cup	115
Unsweetened	1/2 cup	50
Apricots		
Raw (12 per pound)	3 apricots	55
Canned, with heavy syrup	1/2 cup	110
Apricot nectar, canned	1/2 cup	75
Avocado, raw (10 ounces)	1 avocado	370
Banana, medium (6 inches)	1 banana	85
Blueberries	1 cup	90
Cherries	10 cherries	45
Cranberry juice cocktail, sweetened	1/2 cup	85
Dates	10 dates	220
Fruit cocktail, canned in heavy syrup	1/2 cup	100
Grapefruit (3¾-inch diameter, about; 1 pound, 1 ounce)	1/2 medium	50
Grapefruit juice, unsweetened	1/2 cup	50
Grapes	10 grapes	40
Grape juice	1/2 cup	85
Cantaloupe (5-inch diameter, 2⅓ pound)	1/2 of fruit	80
Honeydew melon (6½-inch diameter, 5¼ pound)	1/10	50
Orange (2⅝-inch diameter, 2½ per pound)	1 orange	65
Orange juice, unsweetened	1/2 cup	60
Peaches		
Fresh (4 per pound)	1 peach	40
Canned, sweetened	1/2 cup	100
Canned in water	1/2 cup	40
Frozen, sweetened	1/2 cup	110
Pears		
Fresh	1 pear	100
Canned in syrup	1/2 cup	100
Pineapple		
Fresh, diced	1/2 cup	40
Canned in heavy syrup	1/2 cup	95
Pineapple juice, unsweetened	1/2 cup	70
Plums		
Fresh (6½ per pound)	1 plum	30
Canned in heavy syrup	1/2 cup	110
Prunes		
Dried, uncooked (softenized with pits)	5 large	110

Fruit (cont.)	Amount	Calories
Cooked, unsweetened	1/2 cup	130
Prune juice	1/2 cup	100
Raisins	1 ounce, or 3 tablespoons	80
Raspberries	1/2 cup	35
Strawberries	1/2 cup	30
Tangerine (2⅜ inch diameter, 4 per pound)	1 tangerine	40
Tangerine juice, sweetened	1/2 cup	65

Grain Products

	Amount	Calories
Bagel (3-inch diameter)	1 bagel	165
Biscuits (2-inch diameter)	1 biscuit	100
Boston brown bread (3¼ × ½ inches)	1 slice	95
Cracked wheat bread (18 slices per pound loaf)	1 slice	65
French bread (5 × 2½ × 1 inches)	1 slice	100
Italian bread (4½ × 3¼ × ¾ inches)	1 slice	85
Raisin bread (18 slices per loaf)	1 slice	65
Rye bread (4¾ × 3¾ × 7/16 inches)	1 slice	60
Pumpernickel (5 × 4 × ⅜ inches)	1 slice	80
White bread		
Firm crumb (20 slices per loaf)	1 slice	65
Soft crumb (18 slices per loaf)	1 slice	70
Whole wheat bread		
Firm crumb (18 slices per loaf)	1 slice	60
Soft crumb (16 slices per loaf)	1 slice	65
Breakfast cereals, cooked		
Farina, quick cooking	1 cup	105
Oatmeal	1 cup	130
Wheat		
Rolled	1 cup	180
Whole, meal	1 cup	110
Ready-to-eat cereals (without milk, check individual brands)		
Bran flakes (40% bran)	1 cup	105
Corn flakes	1 cup	95
Oats, puffed, plain	1 cup	100

Grain (cont.)	Amount	Calories
Wheat		
Puffed, plain	1 cup	55
Puffed, presweetened	1 cup	140
Shredded, plain	1 cup	90
Wheat germ	1 tablespoon	25
Bulgur, canned, seasoned	1 cup	245
Angelfood cake (9¾-inch diameter)	1/12 of cake	135
Coffeecake (7¾ × 5⅝ × 1¼ inches)	1/6 of cake	230
Cupcake (2½-inch diameter)		
Plain	1 cupcake	90
Iced	1 cupcake	130
Gingerbread (8 inches square)	1/9 of cake	175
Yellow cake with chocolate icing (8- or 9-inch diamater)	1/16 of cake	235
Pound cake (8½ × 3½ × 3¼ inch)	1/17 of cake	160
Cookies		
Brownies with nuts (1¾ × 1¾ × ⅞ inches)	1 brownie	95
Chocolate chip (2¼-inch diameter × ⅜ inch)	4 cookies	200
Fig bars (1⅝ × 1⅜ × ⅜ inches)	4 cookies	200
Oatmeal with raisins (2⅝-inch diameter × ¼ inch)	4 cookies	235
Sandwich type cookies (1¾-inch diameter × ⅜ inch)	4 cookies	200
Vanilla wafers (1¾-inch diameter × ¼ inch)	10 cookies	185
Crackers		
Graham, plain (2-1/2 inches square)	2 crackers	55
Saltines	4 crackers	50
Rye wafers (1⅞ × 3½ inches)	2 wafers	45
Danish pastry, plain (4¼ inch diameter × 1 inch)	1 pastry	275
Doughnuts, cake type (plain 1½-inch diameter × 1 inch)	1 doughnut	100
Macaroni (cut lengths, elbows, shells)		
Cooked firm	1 cup	190
Cooked tender	1 cup	155
Macaroni and cheese (home recipe)	1 cup	430
Muffins (2⅜ × 1½ inches)		
Bran	1 muffin	105
Corn	1 muffin	125
Noodles		
Egg, cooked	1 cup	200
Chow mein, canned	1 cup	220

Grain (cont.)	Amount	Calories
Pancakes (4-inch diameter)		
Buckwheat from mix	1 cake	55
Plain homemade	1 cake	60
Pies (9-inch diameter)		
Apple	1/7 of pie	345
Banana cream	1/7 of pie	285
Blueberry	1/7 of pie	325
Cherry	1/7 of pie	350
Custard	1/7 of pie	285
Lemon meringue	1/7 of pie	305
Mince	1/7 of pie	365
Peach	1/7 of pie	345
Pecan	1/7 of pie	495
Pumpkin	1/7 of pie	275
Pizza, cheese (12-inch diameter)	1/8 of pizza	145
Popcorn		
With salt and oil	1 cup	40
Plain	1 cup	25
Sugar coated	1 cup	135
Pretzel sticks (2¼ inches long)	10 sticks	10
Pretzels, thin twisted (3¼ × 2¼ × ¼ inches)	10 pretzels	235
Rice, white, cooked		
Long grain	1 cup	225
Parboiled	1 cup	185
Rolls		
Frankfurter and hamburger (8 per 11½ ounce package)	1 roll	120
Hard (3¾-inch diameter, 2 inches high)	1 roll	155
Hoagie, or submarine (11½ × 3 × 2½ inches)	1 roll	390
Cloverleaf, homemade (2½-inch diameter, 2 inches high)	1 roll	120
Spaghetti		
Cooked firm	1 cup	190
Cooked tender	1 cup	155
Toaster pastries	1 pastry	200
Waffles (7-inch diameter)	1 waffle	210

Legumes (dry), Nuts, Seeds: Related Products	Amount	Calories
Almonds, shelled		
Chopped	1 cup	775
Slivered, not pressed down	1 cup	690
Beans, dry, cooked, drained		
Great Northern	1 cup	210
Pea (navy)	1 cup	225
Beans, canned (solids and liquid)		
White, with		
Frankfurters, sliced	1 cup	365
Pork and tomato sauce	1 cup	310
Pork and sweet sauce	1 cup	385
Red kidney	1 cup	260
Lima beans, cooked, drained	1 cup	260
Blackeye peas, dry, cooked (with residual cooking liquid)	1 cup	190
Brazil nuts, shelled (6 or 8 large)	1 ounce	185
Cashew nuts, roasted in oil	1 cup	785
Hazelnuts, chopped	1 cup	730
Peanuts, roasted in oil	1 cup	840
Peanut butter	1 level tablespoon	95
Pecans, chopped or pieces	1 cup	810
Walnuts		
English, chopped	1 cup	780
Black, chopped	1 cup	785
Lentils, whole, cooked	1 cup	210

Sugar and Sweets

	Amount	Calories
Cake icings		
Boiled white		
Plain	1 cup	295
With coconut	1 cup	605
Uncooked chocolate made with milk and butter	1 cup	1035
Creamy fudge from mix and water	1 cup	830
White	1 cup	1200
Candy		
Caramels, plain or chocolate	1 ounce	115
Chocolate, semisweet, pieces	1 cup	860
Chocolate, milk, plain	1 ounce	145
Fondant, uncoated	1 ounce	105
Chocolate-coated peanuts	1 ounce	160
Fudge, chocolate, plain	1 ounce	115

Sweets (cont.)	Amount	Calories
Gum drops	1 ounce	100
Hard	1 ounce	110
Marshmallows	1 ounce	90
Chocolate-flavored beverage powders (about 4 heaping teaspoons per ounce)	1 ounce	100
Honey	1 tablespoon	65
Jams and preserves	1 tablespoon	55
Jellies	1 tablespoon	50
Syrups		
Chocolate-flavored syrup or topping		
Thin type	2 tablespoons	90
Fudge type	2 tablespoons	125
Molasses, cane, light	1 tablespoon	50
Sorghum	1 tablespoon	55
Table blended, chiefly corn, light and dark	1 tablespoon	60
Sugar		
Brown, pressed down	1 cup	820
White, granulated	1 cup	770
White, granulated	1 tablespoon	45
Powdered, sifted	1 cup	385

Vegetables and Vegetable Products

	Amount	Calories
Asparagus spears, cooked (½-inch diameter at base)		
Fresh	4 spears	10
Frozen	4 spears	15
Canned	4 spears	15
Beans		
Lima, frozen, cooked		
Fordhook	1 cup	170
Baby limas	1 cup	210
Snap or green, cooked, drained		
Fresh	1 cup	30
Frozen, cuts and French style	1 cup	35
Canned, drained solids	1 cup	30
Yellow or wax, cooked and drained		
Fresh	1 cup	30
Frozen	1 cup	35
Canned, drained solids	1 cup	30
Bean sprouts (mung)		
Fresh	1 cup	35
Cooked, drained	1 cup	35

Vegetables (cont.)	Amount	Calories
Beets		
Cooked, drained, peeled		
Whole beets (2-inch diameter)	2 beets	30
Diced or sliced	1 cup	55
Canned, drained		
Whole beets, small	1 cup	60
Diced or sliced	1 cup	65
Beet greens (leaves and stems cooked), drained	1 cup	25
Blackeye peas, cooked and drained		
Fresh	1 cup	180
Frozen	1 cup	220
Broccoli, cooked, drained		
Fresh stalk, medium size	1 stalk	45
Fresh stalks, cut into 1/2-inch pieces	1 cup	40
Frozen		
Stalk	1 stalk	10
Chopped	1 cup	50
Brussels sprouts, cooked		
Fresh	1 cup	55
Frozen	1 cup	50
Cabbage		
Raw, shredded or chopped	1 cup	20
Cooked, drained	1 cup	30
Carrots (7½ inches × 1⅛ inches, about 18 strips)		
Raw	1 carrot	30
Grated	1 cup	45
Cooked, crosswise cut, drained	1 cup	50
Canned, sliced, drained	1 cup	45
Cauliflower		
Raw, chopped	1 cup	30
Cooked, drained		
Fresh flower buds	1 cup	30
Frozen flowerets	1 cup	30
Celery, raw (8 × 1½ inches at root end)	1 stalk	5
Collards, cooked, drained		
Fresh leaves without stems	1 cup	65
Frozen, chopped	1 cup	50
Corn, sweet, cooked and drained		
Ear		
Fresh (5 × 1¾ inches)	1 ear	70
Frozen (5 inches)	1 ear	120
Kernels		
Frozen	1 cup	130

Vegetables (cont.)

	Amount	Calories
Canned, creamed	1 cup	210
Canned, vacuum pack	1 cup	175
Canned, wet pack, drained	1 cup	140
Cucumbers, slices (⅛ inch thick)		
Large (2⅛-inch diameter)	6 slices	5
Small (1¾-inch diameter)	8 slices	5
Dandelion greens, cooked, drained	1 cup	35
Endive, curly, chicory or escarole raw, cut into small pieces	1 cup	10
Kale, cooked (leaf only)	1 cup	45
Salad greens, chopped	1 cup	10
Mushrooms, raw, sliced or chopped	1 cup	20
Mustard greens, cooked and drained (leaf only)	1 cup	30
Okra pods, cooked (3 × ⅝ inches)	10 pods	30
Onions, raw		
Chopped	1 cup	65
Sliced	1 cup	45
Onions, cooked, whole or sliced, drained	1 cup	60
Parsnips, cooked, diced, or 2-inch lengths	1 cup	100
Peas, green		
Canned, whole, drained	1 cup	150
Frozen, cooked, drained	1 cup	110
Peppers, sweet, raw or cooked (5 per pound) stem and seeds removed	1 pod	15
Potatoes		
Baked, peeled after baking (2 per pound)	1 potato	145
Boiled (3 per pound)		
Peeled before boiling	1 potato	105
Peeled after boiling	1 potato	90
French fried, strip (2 to 3½ inches long)		
Fresh	10 strips	135
Frozen, oven heated	10 strips	110
Hash brown, frozen	1 cup	345
Mashed		
Fresh, with milk	1 cup	135
Fresh with milk and butter	1 cup	195
Dehydrated flakes with water, milk, butter and salt	1 cup	195
Potato chips (1¾ × 2½ inch oval cross section)	10 chips	115
Potato salad, with cooked dressing	1 cup	250

Vegetables (cont.)

	Amount	Calories
Pumpkin, canned	1 cup	80
Radishes, raw	4 radishes	5
Sauerkraut, canned (solids and liquid)	1 cup	40
Spinach		
Raw, chopped	1 cup	15
Cooked, drained		
Fresh	1 cup	40
Frozen, chopped	1 cup	45
Canned, leaf	1 cup	50
Squash, cooked		
Summer, diced, drained	1 cup	30
Winter, baked or mashed	1 cup	130
Sweet potato (fresh 5 × 2 inches about 2½ per pound)		
Baked in skin, peeled	1 potato	160
Boiled in skin, peeled	1 potato	170
Candied (2½ × 2-inch pieces)	1 piece	175
Canned		
Solid pack (mashed)	1 cup	275
Vacuum pack (2¾ × 1 inch)	1 piece	45
Tomatoes		
Fresh 2⅗-inch diameter (4 ounces)	1 tomato	25
Canned (liquid and solids)	1 cup	20
Tomato catsup	1 tablespoon	15
	1 cup	290
Tomato juice, canned	1 cup	45
Turnips, cooked, diced	1 cup	35
Turnip greens, cooked, drained	1 cup	30
Vegetables, mixed, frozen, cooked	1 cup	115

Miscellaneous Items

Barbecue sauce	1 cup	230
Beverages, alcoholic		
Beer	12 fl. ounces	150
Gin, rum, vodka, whiskey		
80 proof	1-1/2 fl. ounces	95
86 proof	1-1/2 fl. ounces	105
90 proof	1-1/2 fl. ounces	110
Wine		
Dessert	3-1/2 fl. ounces	140
Table	3-1/2 fl. ounces	85
Beverages, non-alcoholic, carbonated, sweetened		
Carbonated water	12 fl. ounces	115
Cola	12 fl. ounces	145

Miscellaneous (cont.)	Amount	Calories
Fruit-flavored sodas and Tom Collins mixer	12 fl. ounces	170
Ginger ale	12 fl. ounces	115
Root beer	12 fl. ounces	150
Chocolate, bitter or baking	1 ounce	145
Gelatin, dry (7 grams)	1 envelope	25
Gelatin dessert, prepared with gelatin dessert powder and water	1 cup	140
Mustard, prepared yellow	1 teaspoon	5
Olive, pickled, canned		
Green	4 medium	15
Ripe	3 small	15
Pickles, cucumber		
Dill (3¾ inches × 1¼ inches in diameter)	1 pickle	5
Sweet, gherkin, small (2½ × ¾ inches)	1 pickle	20
Relish, finely chopped, sweet	1 tablespoon	20
Popsicle, 3 fl. ounce size	1 popsicle	70
Soups, canned, condensed		
Prepared with equal amounts of milk		
Cream of chicken	1 cup	180
Cream of mushroom	1 cup	215
Tomato	1 cup	175
Prepared with equal amounts of water		
Bean with pork	1 cup	170
Beef broth, bouillon, consommé	1 cup	30
Beef noodle	1 cup	65
Clam chowder (Manhattan)	1 cup	80
Cream of chicken	1 cup	95
Cream of mushroom	1 cup	135
Minestrone	1 cup	105
Split pea	1 cup	145
Tomato	1 cup	90
Vegetable beef	1 cup	80
Vegetarian	1 cup	80
Dehydrated soup mixes		
Unprepared		
Onion (½-ounce package)	1 package	150
Prepared with water		
Chicken noodle	1 cup	55
Onion	1 cup	35
Tomato vegetable with noodle	1 cup	65

Miscellaneous (cont.)	Amount	Calories
Vinegar, cider	1 tablespoon	trace
White sauce, medium	1 cup	405

Note. Additional information can be found in "The Nutritive Value of Foods," which can be ordered from the U.S. Government Printing Office (see "Recommended Reading").

The Awful Truth

Here's a summary of some really high risk foods for gaining weight if they are eaten in addition to the calories allowed to hold to the correct weight for those over fifty. These figures are calculated on the basis of one pound of body fat being equal to 3,500 calories. If you eat 100 calories extra per day per year, expect a weight gain of about 10 pounds; if 150 calories extra per day, expect about a 15 pound weight gain at the end of the year; if 200 calories extra per day, a weight gain of 20 pounds a year may be expected!

When a person eats the following foods per day per year over what is needed to maintain normal weight, the weight gain is as follows:

Food Eaten Daily	Weight Gain per Year
4 chocolate chip cookies, 2½-inch diameter (200 calories)	About 20 pounds
10 potato chips (115 calories)	About 12 pounds
1 doughnut 2½-inch diameter, 1 inch high	About 10 pounds
3 level teaspoons sugar	About 4½ pounds
1 level tablespoon honey	About 6½ pounds
1 level tablespoon peanut butter	About 9½ pounds
1 cupcake, 2½-inch diameter	About 13 pounds

Check your favorite snacks! It pays to figure out how many extra calories they may be costing you over your needs!

11
Constipation and Other Problems

CONSTIPATION IS A CURSE of the after-fifty years. Nearly everyone in our Feel-Better Group was troubled by it. A good number, but not all, were greatly helped by making changes in their life style and diet.

Constipation is not simple. It has many causes and complications. Because it may be the sign of a serious disturbance in the body, it should always be checked by a doctor.

What Is Normal?

For comfort and good health, most people do best with a daily bowel movement. Others empty the bowels every second or third day, and feel just as good. Rare individuals empty the bowels at even longer intervals, and still feel comfortable. A regular pattern, or rhythm, is the important thing in bowel movements.

Here are a dozen most common causes of constipation. They may help to pinpoint special constipation problems.

1. Other disorders in the body
2. Bad food habits

A diet may be too low in bulk; or too high in very refined foods; or too low in fats; or lacking in the nutrients that the body must have to work well.

3. Not enough water, or other liquids, during the day
4. Abuse in use of laxatives or enemas
5. Eating at odd hours, no set mealtimes
6. Poor toilet habits

For example, a repeated lack of response to the urge to have a bowel movement. Some people avoid a bowel movement because they have painful hemorrhoids, fissures, or a hard fecal mass. A doctor should be consulted to correct these conditions.

7. Obstructions

These may be adhesions or kinks in the intestine, caused by scar tissue from an operation, tension, pressure, etc.

8. Undue tension

Almost everyone suffers from this in modern life. Getting it under control often reduces constipation.

9. Over-stimulation

This may be due to introducing irritating foods into the system. For instance, for some people, it may be an overuse of bran, or other foods. Or the overstimulation may come from excitement such as that of attending a football game, followed by a party, and a long trip home.

10. Overtaxing the body's strength
11. Lack of exercise

Without exercise, there is weakness in the sketetal muscles and poor tone of the intestinal muscle. The intestinal muscle becomes flabby like a shriveled balloon and cannot work well.

12. Change in usual activity

For example, many people on vacation change their routine and eat their meals at different times from at home. This may cause constipation in some individuals.

Three Main Types of Constipation

The most common form of constipation is what doctors call atonic, or habitual, constipation. Because the intestinal walls lack the right muscular control, the body is not able to propel or move a digested mass of food through at a normal rate. When this happens, the food stands longer than it should in the large intestine. The bacteria in the food remain in contact longer with the intestinal walls. This causes digestive disturbances such as gas and pain. When the diet is made up of too highly refined foods, not enough roughage or bulk gets to the intestinal tract to stimulate the muscle to pass the food through the body and get rid of waste.

Another form of constipation is spastic constipation. It may be present by itself, or in association with a disease. It is the opposite of atonic constipation. The intestinal muscle has too much tightness instead of too little, and digested food moves in very irregular patterns. This causes acute pain. Any irritation to the intestinal tract or extreme tension or pressure can cause this condition. When the muscle in the colon, or intestinal tract, is too tense, the digested food mass becomes impacted. The stools are usually small, dry, ribbonlike and often a mucouslike substance is present.

The third type of constipation results from an obstruction in the intestinal tract, such as a kink or adhesions. As a rule, the obstruction requires medical attention. People in this condition are placed on a special diet. Its purpose is not to correct the problem but to keep the body nourished. The diet is usually free from residue, allowing the food to trickle past the obstruction and furnish some of the nutrients needed.

What Can Be Done about Constipation?

When the constipation is related to poor diet and living habits, a lot can be done to correct it.

The most important change to make is to get regularity, routine, into life. The body is a very conservative machine. It does not react well to frequent changes of daily schedule.

Here are some very simple things that can help to free people from this type of constipation:

Take regular, light exercise every day. Walking is ideal.

Take up good toilet habits. Try to go to the toilet at the same time every day. Allow enough time. Never hurry. Sit down in the bathroom and relax. Arrange for whatever puts you in a pleasant mood: listening to music; reading the paper; thinking about favorite things. Take a slightly stooped-over position. This helps the muscles in the intestine to work properly. Placing a small footstool or low box under the feet often helps to put a person in the correct position, especially for very short people. In the ideal position for a bowel movement, the base of the spine is slightly lower than the knees.

Drink more water. A glass or two of plain, warm water before breakfast is very helpful in relieving constipation. Some get the same result with cool water. Most people do not drink enough water for good elimination. The average person should have 6 to 8 cups of water or other liquid a day. Take water between meals. Remember, it is impossible to have normal bowel movements without enough liquid.

Eat meals at the same time every day. People who would overcome constipation must have a regular mealtime schedule. Sit down to eat. Make food time as relaxed and pleasant as possible. Chew thoroughly. Many older people gulp their food. This often triggers a spastic reaction in the intestine.

Try to cut down the tension in life. We all have problems and we all have hard situations that must be handled each day. The challenge is to learn how to handle the problems without getting upset. This is probably the best of all ways to overcome constipation. We admit it's easier said than done, but keep working on it to deal with constipation effectively.

Eat foods that help. Members of the Feel-Better Group who changed their diet to overcome constipation found it quite easy to do. It was a joy to see what a difference it made in their lives. The basic diet problem is that most people eat too many processed foods. These don't give the bulk or fiber that the intestine needs to do its work and push the waste out. Take a look at the meals you have been eating. Do you eat whole wheat bread and breakfast cereals? Fresh fruits and vegetables? Dried beans and peas? If the answer is no, it's a safe guess that constipation may be a problem.

Every day, have some fruits and vegetables, as recommended in the Daily Food Guide. Eat them both raw and cooked to add important fiber to the diet. Especially helpful are leafy vegetables like kale, spinach, escarole, chicory, cabbage. All the fruits help with the problem of constipation. Include dried fruits, too, such as figs, raisins, prunes, etc.

As emphasized, for good nutrition, you need at least four servings of bread and cereals a day. These are just as urgently required for good elimination because of their fiber content. Include some breads and cereals that are whole grain rather than only white breads made from refined flour, or cereals made only from highly refined grains. In an average day's meals, two slices of whole grain bread, a portion of whole grain cereal, and a serving of rice, noodles, or macaroni, or another slice of bread, give important amounts of roughage to help regular bowel movements.

Bran and bran cereals are often eaten to give additional bulk to the diet to help overcome constipation. Be careful not to use too much. It can sometimes cause a bran bolus (a large round mass in the intestine like a ball) that actually obstructs the bowel. This is an example of a good and important food that can cause distress in the body when overused.

For persons who are very sensitive to roughage or fiber in the diet, too much roughage can cause digestive discomfort. If this happens repeatedly, the person should cut down on the amount of high fiber food, and consult a doctor before making any further changes in the kinds of food eaten.

Include fats in the diet. A proper amount of fats in the diet is very helpful to those who are constipated. (See chapter 7, "The Handy Food Finder," for correct amounts.) An excess amount of fat, however, can cause diarrhea, or diarrhea alternating with spastic constipation.

Include two or more servings of protein foods. These foods are needed for the normal working of the body although not for bulk.

Many people have heard that milk is constipating. This is not so when a balanced diet is eaten. Everyone after fifty should have two cups of milk a day. It is only when milk and meat are used as the main foods in the diet, and most other foods are left out, that there may be a problem.

A word about laxatives. When a person has used an excessive amount of laxatives or enemas to relieve constipation, the muscles in the lower bowel may be affected in a way that cannot be reversed. Although eating a diet with enough, or with extra, bulk may be of some help, it is almost impossible to correct this condition altogether. Often, because of this change in the lower bowel, the use of laxatives must be continued. In this case, it is very important to consult a doctor to find out which type of laxative will be most helpful without doing further harm.

If a laxative must be taken, be sure to use it as far from mealtimes as possible. Otherwise, the laxative may carry the food through the body in too short a time for the body to absorb the nutrients in the food before it is eliminated.

Mineral oil is not the best choice in a laxative unless prescribed by a doctor. It carries away the fat-soluble vitamins, and the body does not have a chance to use them.

The relief of constipation is a sure way for people after fifty to feel better. We hope that some of these ideas may help.

12
The Feel-Better Kitchen: How to Plan for It

A lot of things go on in the feel-better kitchen that don't go on in other people's kitchens.

There is the crunch and crackle of crisp green salads, the glow and beauty of fresh fruit, and there are little treats in the cupboard and refrigerator to give a lift to life. These are good-for-you goodies, not loaded with sugar, salt, and fat.

Maybe you, like the Feel-Better Group, are saying: "Oh, I can never have these foods because they come in packages too big for a person living alone." We'll show you how to get around that. Or you may be saying, as they did: "I simply haven't the time." Well, it does take a little time to eat well. There are a few fix-ahead things to do each week.

But look at it this way. In little more time than it takes at the beauty parlor, you can do all your fix-ahead work for feel-better food for a whole week! Many women don't feel their best without a regular shampoo and set. That makes them feel good inside about their outside. Setting aside a feel-better food time each week makes a person feel good inside, and it shows up outside, too, in a more attractive appearance. Men, too, who live alone can borrow some time from a busy life to do this important work each week. It won't take them any more time than it does to wash and polish a car. This small investment of time and effort can make the difference, as it did for our Feel-Better Group members, between a tired, low-spirited individual and a peppy, lively one.

Plan for feel-better food fixing time early in the morning, or late at night, whatever your way of life, and it will reward you in many ways—better health, more variety, and much more pleasure. These feel-better kitchen tips will help you see your way to eating at its best.

Fix-Ahead Raw Vegetables

The nippy textures, the racy, earthy flavors of raw vegetables make a great change of pace in the day's food. A natural source of vitamins, minerals, and roughage, they're important to eat daily for good health—and their calorie count is very low! Raw vegetables make an ideal snack but we've found that unless people keep raw vegetables ready to eat in the refrigerator, they don't make a habit of snacking on them. So let's try the fix-ahead way to have these great snacks ready to eat.

Ready-to-Eat Carrot Sticks

Carrots are an excellent source of vitamin A and they are easy to fix ahead. When buying carrots, choose those that are stiff and relatively clean; never soft and flexible. It's better to buy small carrots. Larger ones are tougher and may have woody centers so they have to be thrown away.

Clean the carrots by covering them with cold water and scrubbing them, if needed. Peel or scrape, if desired. Remove tip and base.

Place a carrot on a firm surface and cut it in half lengthwise. Now place cut side down. Cut the carrot lengthwise into the thinnest sticks possible. It may surprise you to discover that when carrots are cut very thin, even people who have trouble chewing can usually manage them.

To store. Moisten a white paper towel, wrap the carrot sticks in it, and place in a plastic bag, or in a plastic or other tightly covered container. Store in the refrigerator. If the towel dries out, just add a few drops of water to it and rewrap the carrot sticks. These sticks should keep for four or five days.

Try making carrot sticks from one medium size carrot or two small ones. If this meets your snack needs, fine. You may want to make more at a time when you get the carrot snacking habit. True, there is some vitamin loss in preparing and storing carrots this way but it is better than doing without them altogether because they are not ready to eat when you feel like them.

Those who feel they can trust themselves to make carrot sticks a few at a time can have the carrots washed and ready, stored as above, and cut off each day just the number of sticks desired.

People who have chewing problems can still enjoy raw carrots by grating them instead of cutting them into sticks. Use an old-fashioned flat metal grater, or any kind on hand, or put the carrots through the coarse blade of a food grinder, if available. Store the grated carrots in a small glass jar, place a moist white paper towel on top, then a piece of waxed paper or foil so moisture will not be lost, and cover with a tight lid. Store in refrigerator. Check to be sure paper towel stays moist.

Besides their use as snack, grated carrots are wonderful to keep on hand to make meals more nourishing and interesting. Use these carrots as a vitamin A booster in a salad, or as part of a soup, or in a tomato sauce, or in any mixed casserole, or as a colorful garnish. Grated carrots are good in homemade cookies, too.

Ready-to-Eat Green or Red Pepper Sticks

When buying green or red peppers, choose those that are firm and fleshy. Flabby peppers or those with very thin walls or spots have already started to spoil and good vitamins have been lost.

Wash the pepper, cut in half, take out seeds and white part. Pat the pepper dry thoroughly; peppers start to spoil immediately in high humidity. Cut the pepper lengthwise into the thinnest possible sticks. Store the same as for carrots. Some may prefer to use half the pepper for sticks; the other half for seasoning in cooking.

Many other vegetables are enjoyable raw as snacks and in salads. Try zucchini, cauliflower, broccoli, asparagus. Cut in small pieces and store as above.

Planning for Fresh Fruit

Fruits belong in the feel-better kitchen. They are part of the poetry of life. The beauty of fruit gladdens the spirit. The zest, the fresh, juicy flavors, give a lift to the dreariest day. And we already know what fruit vitamins, minerals, and fiber do for the body.

Many after-fifty people who like fresh fruit complain that the packages in the store are too large for their use. And they're right. They buy the fruit, only to have it spoil. The next time you buy fresh fruit and you want less than the amount that is packaged, go to the store manager. Ask him to split the package for you. Did you know that in some stores there have been so many complaints about prepackaged fruit that they now have fresh fruit loose in any amount that people want to buy, as well as prepackaged? If enough people ask a store manager to sell fruit so that anyone can buy the amount needed, no matter how little, the change will be made. After all, your money is as good as anyone else's. People over fifty make up nearly 25 percent of the population. That accounts for a large amount of the money spent in stores. Use your rights to get the feel-better food you need. There's strength in "number power."

The best rule for getting the most for your fruit dollar is to buy only the amount that will be used between one shopping trip and the next. In general, fruit that is ripe will keep longer if stored in the refrigerator. Some fruits keep best in the hydrator compartment because the temperature and moisture levels are right, but there are exceptions. Seasonal fruits like berries spoil quickly and the moisture level of the hydrator is not good for storing them. Store on a refrigerator shelf instead.

Fruits that come from the store wrapped in plastic or in a plastic bag should be removed from this wrapping right away. It tends to rot some fruit. Sort the fruit and store it, or leave at room temperature, if it is unripe.

Here are a few tips for selecting and storing popular fruits.

Apples

Buy apples that are firm, crisp, and have good color. Never buy apples with wrinkled peel, bruise marks, worm holes, or spoil spots. At home, rinse them and dry them. Place in hydrator of refrigerator. When ready to use, wash apples carefully. Many apples are covered with a thin wax or oil, used to prevent loss of water, so the second washing is important. Depending on freshness at time of buying, apples may be kept in hydrator for at least one week, and often longer.

Bananas

Bananas may be found at the store in any stage of ripeness from green to green-tipped to all-yellow or yellow flecked with brown, the ripest stage of all. For eating immediately, most people prefer the all-yellow peel or yellow flecked with brown. These are the most easily digestible fruit. To ripen bananas at other stages, leave them out at room temperature. However, once they are ripe, as indicated by the peel changing color, they should be stored in the refrigerator, unless they are to be eaten immediately. The peel may turn very dark in the refrigerator but the fruit inside remains good.

When bananas get very ripe, they are delicious to mash and use in a homemade banana bread, in the Feel Better Breakfast in a Drink, page 30, or in another beverage. Sometimes stores will reduce the price of bananas that are very, very ripe. This is a good buy in any quantity that can be used quickly, either to eat out of hand, or to use in a pudding, fresh-fruit cup, or as above.

Peaches and Apricots

Although there are many varieties of peaches, there are two basic kinds, clingstones and freestones. Freestones have softer fruit with fine flavor, and they're good for eating raw or for freezing. Clingstone peaches are known as canning peaches. They are firmer and hold their shape better. Ripe peaches of either kind have a rich, yellow-orange color with patches of red. Peaches should be firm but not hard, without green color. Peaches that are very soft, overripe, or bruised are not good buys.

To store ripe peaches, refrigerate them without washing. Wash only just before eating. Because peaches ripen quickly, it is best to buy only a few at a time. Should more be bought than can be used right away, wash the peaches, peel them, slice, and cook them. Use as a stewed fruit dessert, as a topping on ice cream or pudding, in a pie, or in a "grunt," the old-fashioned dumpling and fruit dessert.

It's best to cook peaches in a very small amount of liquid without sugar. Then taste the cooked peaches, and add sugar if needed. When using a recipe, follow directions but adjust amount of sugar to your taste. You may prefer to reduce directions for a half-cup of sugar to a third-cup. This is your choice for a feel-better diet.

Apricots are picked green for shipping to market. They are, of course, only at their best when ripe so be sure to choose firm apricots with a rich, golden color. Avoid soft, wilted, or shriveled fruit. Apricots spoil fast. Moisture only speeds the spoilage so store the fruit unwashed in the refrigerator. Wash only when ready to use.

Length of Time Fruits Keep in the Refrigerator

Apples, eating, ripe	1 to 2 weeks
Apricots	3 to 5 days
Avocadoes	3 to 5 days
Blackberries	1 or 2 days
Blueberries	3 to 5 days
Cherries	1 to 2 days
Cranberries	1 to 2 weeks
Figs	1 to 2 days
Grapes	3 to 5 days
Peaches	3 to 5 days
Pears	3 to 5 days
Raspberries	1 to 2 days
Strawberries	1 to 2 days
Watermelon	2 to 5 days

Referring to this little chart may help to decide what amounts you can buy without waste from spoilage.

More than one of our Feel-Better Group friends told us "But I can't afford fresh fruit, it's so expensive." "Do you buy doughnuts?" we asked. "Yes." "Potato chips?" "Yes." "Candy bars?" "Yes." "Well, for the price of a couple of doughnuts, and for less than the cost of a bag of potato chips, or a candy bar, you can buy one or more fresh apples or oranges, or other fruits in season. You *can* afford fresh fruit but it's a choice. That's what feel-better food is all about!"

Planning for Vitamin C Foods

Frozen Orange Juice Concentrate

This product is often an excellent buy for vitamin C but our feel-better people complained that it comes in too large a size for them to use up in a reasonable time. Together, we worked out a good solution to this problem. Here it is:

While the orange concentrate is still frozen, open the container at both ends. Push one end of the concentrate out a little. With a kitchen knife, cut off just the amount needed to make the quantity of juice desired. For example, a 6-ounce container of frozen orange juice concentrate makes up to 24 ounces. When you want a half-cup serving (4 ounces), just push out the frozen juice and cut off one-sixth of the total package. Cover ends of opened container tightly with aluminum foil or plastic wrap. Return frozen portion to the freezer. Place the amount of concentrate removed in a measuring cup and fill to the half-cup mark with cold water. Stir well and use. For the 12-ounce container, cut off one-twelfth and follow directions as above.

If your freezing compartment in the refrigerator does not keep orange juice concentrate frozen solid, just spoon it out in the amount above, and add water.

Oranges and Grapefruit

These, like frozen orange juice concentrate, are one of the richest natural sources of vitamin C.

Buy oranges and grapefruit that are heavy for their size. Avoid fruit with bruised, cut, soft, or pitted peel. Incidentally, strict state regulations require fruit to be tree-ripened. The slightly greenish color or russeting (splotches) on the peel of certain varieties of citrus fruit does not affect the quality or the flavor. Bright-colored fruit may have color added but not necessarily.

Citrus fruit may be kept for a few days at room temperature. It will keep better in the refrigerator. However, if held too long at cold temperature, the peel may become pitted and the flesh inside the orange may discolor. Try to buy oranges and grapefruit in amounts which can be used within a week to ten days.

Strawberries

These are high in vitamin C, as noted in the Food Finder. A half-cup of strawberries meets the vitamin C need for the day so when they are in season, you may want to get your "C" this way.

Buy berries with the stem and caps attached. They should appear fresh, of uniform color, and firm but not hard. Avoid berries that are green or bruised or spoiled. Watch for mildew.

To store, refrigerate berries without washing until shortly before serving time. If the fruit is wet, it starts to spoil.

For additional information about buying and storing fresh fruits, see appendix, "Recommended Reading."

Cabbage

As you know, cabbage is a good vitamin C food. When buying, look for firm, fresh, well-colored heads. The more green color in the leaves, the more goodness and flavor in the cabbage. Avoid heads that are yellow.

To store, remove spoiled parts of leaves, wash under running water, drain off or dry the head. Store in tightly closed plastic bag. Well-chosen cabbage, properly stored, keeps for two or more weeks in the refrigerator.

Those who do not have room to store a whole cabbage, or do not want to eat cabbage that often, can ask the produce man to cut a head in half or into smaller portions.

To keep the vitamin C in raw cabbage, cut or shred it only just before ready to serve or cook.

Potatoes

Many people do not realize that potatoes can give a good amount of vitamin C to a meal though not the total need for the day in a single serving.

Buy potatoes that have no cuts, bruises, decayed spots, sprouts, or green color. The green color is solanin, which forms when potatoes are stored in the light at too low a temperature. Solanin causes bitter flavor. It may also be toxic if eaten in large amounts. Should potatoes have green color, cut out the green part when preparing them.

New potatoes usually have thin skins that separate from the potatoes when cooked. They are best for boiling and for creaming.

Potatoes should be stored in a cool, dark, dry place, away from light, and with good ventilation. When stored at a temperature of from 45° to 50° F., potatoes may be held for several months. In apartments or homes where it is warm, potatoes keep for only a week or two.

Do not store potatoes in the refrigerator. The potato starch turns to sugar. When this happens, the potatoes turn brown when fried and they become gummy when mashed or baked.

Planning for Dark Green Leafy Vegetables

Since green "leafies" are needed in the diet at least every other day to help the body to work well, it's important to plan for them. For people who live alone, this isn't easy.

Friends tell us that greens such as spinach, kale, turnip greens and mustard greens, and collards are often not available in their markets except in frozen form. This is a problem but it can be handled.

If you can get spinach fresh, usually in plastic bags, you can use it up nicely in three or four days by varying the way it is served in your meals. Have you ever tried a salad made with uncooked spinach leaves? It's so delicious that gourmet restaurants feature it at a fancy price. Raw spinach leaves can be used, too, in place of lettuce in a sandwich, or to make a Spinach and Egg-Fry (recipe on page 194). Cook some of the spinach, serving half hot for dinner, refrigerate the rest, covered, and serve with your favorite sauce a day or so later, or use it in a hearty chicken egg-drop soup.

As for the 10-ounce package of frozen spinach or other greens, we have tried every way to divide that package at home, including using a small kitchen saw, and we find that nothing really works. Therefore, one is forced to cook the whole package at one time, and use the cooked greens, carefully stored, at different meals. Since the greens will keep three to four days, this is practical. That is just the time in which a leafy green vegetable should be eaten—every other day.

It's true that vegetables lose vitamins when they are stored after cooking, or reheated. But the choice between a slight loss of vitamins and not having leafy green vegetables at all is an easy one to make in the feel-better diet.

Cooking these greens in the minimum amount of water will help to retain vitamins. And if you store these cooked greens well, you will cut down the vitamin loss, too. When you reheat greens, do it quickly, and eat them at once, to avoid vitamin loss.

After cooking, remove the portion you are going to have for dinner, and cool the remaining cooked greens as quickly as possible. Place them in a small container with a tightly fitting lid. The container should allow for the very least amount of air at the top because the vitamins are kept in the food better that way. Should you have any cooking liquid left, don't pour it away. Store it with the greens. Remember that the water-soluble vitamins are in that liquid. Refrigerate immediately. Never let greens stand around in the kitchen after cooking. The sooner they get into the refrigerator after cooking, the better they will keep the nutrients they have, and food spoilage will also be avoided.

Those who can't find fresh spinach and who don't want to cook frozen spinach and serve it more than once, might prefer canned spinach. Heat only the amount to be used at one meal, and store the rest, properly covered, in the refrigerator, to be served in another meal.

Other Vegetables

People tell us they often buy very small amounts of vegetables, either fresh, frozen, or canned. As for the frozen vegetables, it's sometimes better to buy the bigger size packages (20 ounces) in the plastic bags than the 10 ounce boxes, if you have a fairly good size freezing compartment in your refrigerator. The bagged frozen vegetables are much easier to use in small servings. Just take the bag, scrunch it back and forth in your hands, and you can pour out the amount that you want to cook for one meal. The rest can be kept frozen.

Some of the 10-ounce boxes of frozen vegetables, such as peas, lima beans, corn, peas and carrots, and mixed vegetables, can be scrunched and divided into individual portions, too. However, as pointed out, this will not work with frozen greens.

Fix-Ahead Salad Makings

Fresh green salads are so important to good health, the makings should be ready to use in the refrigerator at all times. They contribute vitamins, minerals, and important roughage, not to mention the sheer joy of salad in a meal.

If you can possibly help it, don't be a one-green salad maker. Some people never use any salad green but crisp head iceberg lettuce, but there are so many other salad greens to enjoy. There's romaine lettuce with long, tapering leaves. There's escarole, a loose-leaved head, white at the base, dark green and ruffled at the tip. There's a slight nip to the taste that is very pleasant in the salad bowl. Chicory, or curly endive, as it is sometimes called, is frilly and fancy-looking. It's good by itself and it looks delightful in a mixed salad. Then there is Boston lettuce, flat-leaved and loose rather than tightly bunched. Those living near farms may find field salad available, a tender, delicious green with small, oval leaves.

Unfortunately, there may not be all these greens available where you live but do look for them, learn to recognize them, and enjoy them for their contrasting tastes and textures when you can get them.

When nutritionists compared crisp head lettuce such as iceberg with escarole, or chicory, they found there is nine times as much vitamin A in equal amounts of these greens as in iceberg lettuce. Remember, the darker green the leaf, the higher the vitamin A! You have only to look at iceberg lettuce to get the message. However, if only iceberg lettuce is sold at your market, use it but add vitamin boosters to improve the nutrition of your salad. These might be a few leaves of fresh spinach, some grated carrot or some green pepper, watercress, or a few dandelion leaves that you might find while taking a walk. Use cooked vitamin A vegetables to boost your salad, too, such as peas, green beans, broccoli, and others.

How to Fix and Store Raw Greens

First, throw away any bruised parts that are wilted or have insect damage. Wash in cold water by moving the salad green back and forth in the water. This will remove any dirt or dust or small insects that may be there. Take the salad greens out of the water and rinse in fresh water a second time. Take the salad greens out of the water and shake well. Allow them to stand in a strainer or your dish rack until most of the water has run out. Moisten a clean dish towel, wrap the salad greens in the dish towel and place in a covered container or a plastic bag. Store in refrigerator.

Don't store greens unwrapped in the hydrator of your refrigerator. It will wilt and spoil in a very short time. There is so much waste because of this practice. When you follow the directions given above, the salad green will be crisp and crunchy, and keep for a longer period of time. Depending upon your refrigerator and how fresh the salad greens were when you bought them, the greens should keep from five to seven days.

Never cut or break up salad greens before storing them. When you do, the salad greens start to spoil, wilt, and become slimy. Cut or break greens only when about to serve, or no more than an hour before dinner; they still must be kept in the refrigerator. Should you decide to fix your salad early, be sure to cover the bowl with a damp towel. This will also help crisp up the salad.

Some greens such as escarole have so much sand at the base of the leaves that they have to be washed when used, in addition to the first preparation for storage. It's wise to allow time for this extra step.

With crisp salad greens ready-prepared, you won't neglect salads in your meals, or some nice crisp leaves in a sandwich in addition to the filling. It takes only a short time just once a week to take this step for feeling better, so plan for it. You'll like it.

Live-Alones Can Enjoy Fresh Broccoli

Because broccoli is such a blockbuster vegetable for good nutrition, we'd like to give some special hints on how to have it in your meals, both frozen and fresh, if you live alone.

With a little trick or two, a 10-ounce package of frozen broccoli spears can be worked into your plans. It can be separated into unthawed servings and served in different ways at different times. Open the package, take a blunt table knife, and poke it between the spears in the middle until they separate into two parts. Take out half the broccoli, wrap it, and return it to the freezer for future meals. Cook the rest of the broccoli. Eat one serving for dinner. Refrigerate the rest to make a salad with French dressing for the next day's meals. Cook the remaining broccoli that you have frozen when you want it for individual dinners, or by the same plan as above. In some areas, frozen chopped broccoli is sold in 20-ounce bags, which eliminates the difficulty of removing one portion. Just scrunch the package and take out the amount desired for a meal.

Many people throw half a bunch of fresh broccoli away because they don't know how to prepare it to get the most from it. That's like throwing half your money in the garbage pail.

It's smart to cook all the broccoli at once, eat some, and freeze individual portions in small packages. It's delicious and very economical. To prepare fresh broccoli, place it all in a container of cold water for about 10 minutes, to remove any small bugs, dust, or soil clinging to the vegetable. Don't add salt. Salt should be restricted in the diet of older people, as already mentioned, and the broccoli will absorb the salt if it is put in the soaking water. Pour off the water; rinse the broccoli quickly with more cold water. Cut off most of the stalk and set it aside. Take off the tender green leaves. Set aside. With a sharp paring knife, peel off the very thin covering on the broccoli stalks. Slice the stalks; cut into circles the way you would carrots. Set alongside the leaves. The bud, or flower part, will now be left. If the outer covering of the stems looks thick and tough, peel this part off. Cut the broccoli in halves or quarters, depending on the size. Cook in about a cup of water, according to the amount of broccoli and the size of the pan, cover, and bring to a boil. Lower heat and cook until the broccoli is half done. Remove all the broccoli from the pan except a portion that you may want for dinner, which can continue cooking till done. If necessary, add more water. Cool the half-cooked broccoli quickly. When convenient, freeze it in individual servings in sturdy plastic bags, or other containers. Make up a serving that includes some of the leaves, the stalk, and the bud portion of the broccoli. We like to cook broccoli in a heavy fry pan with a tight lid. You can lay all the broccoli flat in it, cook it in the minimum time, and it comes out tender-crisp and green.

We found our friends in the Feel-Better Group weren't buying fresh vegetables because they knew only one way to serve them. This caused boredom in their meals. But when they discovered that there were many ways to enjoy the same good food, they began to buy fresh vegetables more often, even a big bunch of broccoli. When the broccoli has been well-kept at the store, it will store well in the refrigerator for four to six days. In that period, you can cook broccoli fresh each time and make such different dishes as broccoli soup, or a stir-fry vegetable with broccoli and onion, or serve broccoli with your favorite sauce, or plain, or baked with sliced chicken and cheese sauce. Both the chicken and the broccoli should be precooked for that delicious dish.

Other Vegetables

As with fresh broccoli, so with other fresh vegetables. You can buy them in the package size available at the store, cook them all at once, and have one portion for supper, freezing the rest in individual packets to use at other times. Or cook all the vegetable at once, store in a container with a tight lid, and have it every other day in a different way.

If you haven't done much freezing of vegetables and want more information, see the appendix, "Recommended Reading," for helpful publications.

Planning for Our Daily Bread

There's always bread on hand in the feel-better kitchen— bread for good hearty taste, for B vitamins, for minerals such as iron, and for fiber.

"I don't keep bread at home anymore because it gets stale before I can eat it. I'm tired of wasting it." So many people living alone say that. We worked out a way to keep bread on hand without waste.

Buy a pound loaf. Divide it in half. Store one half of the loaf, tightly wrapped, at room temperature. Put the other half, tightly wrapped in plastic, in the freezing compartment of the refrigerator. It will keep fresh for one to two weeks. In a regular freezer, it will keep for one to two months. Bread keeps fresher at room temperature than in the refrigerator. However, in humid weather, it is better to store bread in the refrigerator because this protects against mold. With this simple plan, anyone can keep bread on hand to eat daily without waste.

Of course, if you really want wonderful bread, make it

yourself for pleasure, for the sensational aroma while it's baking, and the joy of eating. Easy recipes are on pages 201-202.

Store homemade bread in the same way as above.

Planning for Milk

There's always milk in the feel-better kitchen refrigerator, ready for drinking and for cooking. Whether milk is bought in fluid form, or made up at home from nonfat dry milk, keep it cold. Never let milk stand out on a counter or table because valuable nutrition will be lost, and the keeping quality reduced. This is true of canned milks, too, once they have been opened.

Milk	Storage and Keeping Time
Milk, fluid	
Fresh whole	Refrigerate, covered. For best flavor, use in 3 to 5 days.
Fresh skim	
Made from nonfat dry milk	
Milk, evaporated	
Unopened	Store at room temperature. Use within 6 months.
Opened	Refrigerate, covered. Use in 3 to 5 days.
Milk, sweetened, condensed	
Unopened	Store at room temperature. Use within a few months.
Opened	Refrigerate, covered. Use in 3 to 5 days.
Milk, dry	
Unopened	Store nonfat dry milk at room temperature. Use within a few months. Store dry whole milk in refrigerator. Use within a few weeks.
Liquefied	Store and use as above for fluid milk.

Nonfat dry milk is handy for live-alones. It has fewer calories, no fat, and it means a considerable saving on milk. It's easy to make this milk by just adding water to the powdered product; follow directions on package. If you're not used to the taste of nonfat dry milk, mix half with whole milk for a richer flavor.

Planning for Cheese

Cheese is a valuable, delicious food, yet many people do not store it correctly to keep its goodness for the longest possible time. Generally, cheese dries out and loses flavor and texture when exposed to air, so always keep it in the refrigerator very tightly wrapped in plastic or aluminum foil. If you have a covered cheese dish, that works well, too.

Soft cheeses such as cottage cheese, ricotta, and cream cheese spoil much faster than hard cheeses like Cheddar and Swiss. Soft cheeses should be refrigerated, covered, and used within three to five days.

Generally, hard cheese such as Cheddar, if refrigerated and wrapped in plastic, or in a tightly closed plastic bag, will keep well for a couple of months unless mold develops. If it does, remove the mold, and use the cheese as quickly as possible.

If cheese should dry out and get hard, don't throw it away. Grate it and store it in the refrigerator in a tightly covered jar. Use to top a casserole, or sprinkle over soups or pizza, or add it to meat loaf.

Freezing is not generally recommended for most cheese because it makes it mealy and crumbly. However, small pieces of brick, Cheddar, Edam, Gouda, Swiss, mozzarella, weighing a pound or less, and not more than an inch thick, can be frozen. Where a crumbly texture is desirable in cheese, as in salad or salad dressings, small pieces of bleu, Roquefort, and Gorgonzola can be frozen.

To freeze cheese, wrap it tightly. Freeze quickly at 0° F.

or below. It may be stored for about four months. To use, take cheese out of freezer, thaw slowly in the refrigerator. The freezer compartment of the refrigerator does not reach 0° F. temperature so it is not recommended that cheese be frozen there.

13
The Feel-Better Kitchen: How to Buy for It

You Can Afford Steak

SEVERAL OF OUR FRIENDS in the Feel-Better Group told us how hard it was for them to have red meat with their reduced incomes. They knew they needed it, but they didn't know how they could afford it. We proved to them that they could with the cut-your-own-meat plan.

If that suggests buying a side of beef, we have no such thing in mind. The plan calls for just one cut of meat, a beef chuck blade steak, usually weighing from two to three pounds. This cut is often available, prepackaged, at the supermarket meat counter. If not, the meat man will cut a blade steak for you.

This money-saving meat plan can feed one person four hearty beef meals, including a steak to broil, and a bonus pot of beef broth. Buy one blade chuck beefsteak of good quality. Both of us have bought this cut in New York supermarkets for less than the price of a precut, prepackaged club chuck steak. You get this nice broiling steak right along with the rest of the beef chuck blade steak when you cut it yourself.

In addition to the club steak, you get one chicken steak, one filet steak, a nice amount of beef for stew, besides bones and meat scraps to make beef broth. The savings are tremendous. Our feel-better people figured they could easily save up to $72 a year with this plan, have all the beef they needed in their diet, and the quality was better than if the beef were bought in separate, smaller cuts from the supermarket meat case.

Why is it that you can get so much more meat for your money if you are willing to do a little meat cutting yourself? It's simple. The butcher cuts meat up into smaller pieces for your convenience. You expect to pay him for his work. But he also knows that he'll get a separate profit on each cut of meat so the more cuts there are, the more profit he makes. When you buy a bigger cut of meat and divide it into smaller cuts yourself, you turn the profit situation around. You put the money in your pocket instead of into the meat man's. Fair is fair. At today's prices for food, you've got to know how to beat the game.

A member of our Feel-Better Group who was always one of the first to try a new idea, said, "Wait till you hear my news! I found beef chuck blade steak on sale at my supermarket for only 59 cents a pound. I bought five, cut them up, and now my freezer is full of high quality, delicious beef, including five fine steaks, at less than I ever paid for meat in my life!"

Two things may strike you about this plan. You may feel it is too hard for you to cut up meat, and you may feel you'll have so much meat at one time it will spoil. We'll show you how easy it is to cut the meat up, and how to cook or freeze the individual beef pieces so that you can manage beautifully without wasting a thing.

If you feel a little squeamish about cutting up meat, you'll soon overcome it once you see what fine quality it brings you for so much less money. The cutting will get easier every time you do it until it is just second nature. The feel-better benefits are great—and your pocketbook will feel better, too.

The Feel-Better Kitchen • 151

Four Beef Meals and a Pot of Soup

First, study this diagram of a beef chuck blade steak. You'll see when you have the cut before you that there are natural divisions between the cuts that you can slide your knife along very easily.

Place the steak on a board on a counter or kitchen table with a piece of waxed paper underneath the meat. Have a large piece of waxed paper nearby on which to place the pieces of meat after you cut them. With your sharpest kitchen knife, start cutting up the steak in this order:

1. Cut around area A as marked on the steak diagram. Remove this piece of meat to the waxed paper on the table. This gives you a cut sold separately at the market by such names as chicken steak, sandwich steak, beef butterfly steak, special minute steak, chuck tenderloin steak, chuck tender, chuck top blade steak, boneless, boneless beef petite steak, and others, depending upon the custom of naming cuts in each locality. Next time you are at the supermarket meat counter, go around and locate this cut by whatever name it is called in your town. Notice the price. You'll get a thrill when you realize how much less you are paying for it by cutting it out of a larger cut. As for cooking, chicken steak is very nice to pan-fry.

2. Now cut around area B for a cut best known as filet chuck but also as boneless chuck filet steak, London broil chuck, chuck under plate steak, middle chuck steak, etc. Put that cut on the waxed paper and go on to the next one.

3. Look for area C in the diagram. Find this on your steak. This will give you the relatively high-priced chuck club steak, delicious to broil. This cut is also known as bottom chuck club; his and hers chuck steak; rib chuck steak, etc. This cut sometimes sells for more per pound than the entire beek chuck blade steak.

4. Cut the remaining meat into cubes and you will have very high quality stewing beef, much better than is usually sold under this name, and much cheaper, too. If you don't

FEEL BETTER AFTER 50 FOOD BOOK • 152

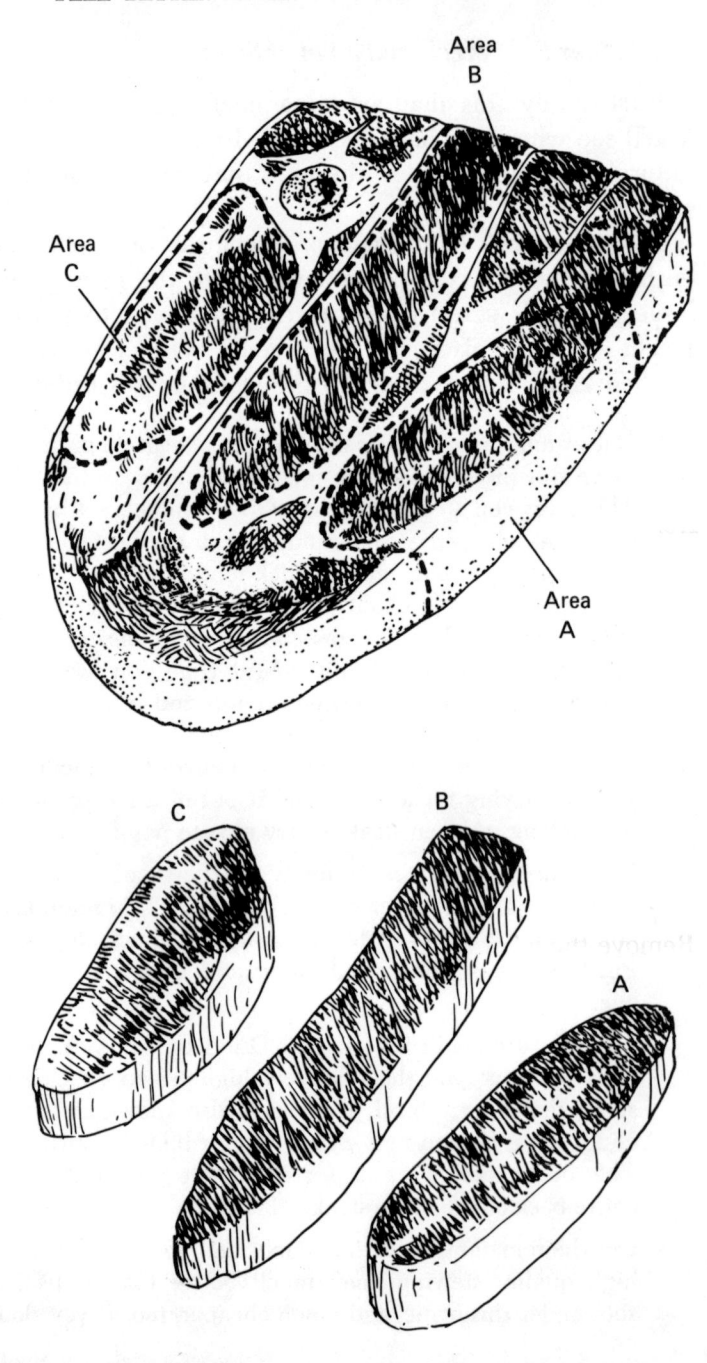

like stew, cut the meat into very thin strips so it will cook quickly on top of the stove. If you have a meat grinder, you can use this beef for chopped beef of very high quality.

5. Use the bones and scraps of meat that are left to make a nourishing beef broth.

If there is more than one person to feed at your house, just buy one beef chuck blade steak per person, and proceed as above for each steak.

How to Make Beef Broth

Place in a large pan that has a tight-fitting lid, the bones from cutting up a chuck steak, or from other beef cuts, and the scraps of meat found in the fat. Depending upon the amount of bones, add from 1 to 2½ quarts of water. Usually the bones from one steak take about 1 quart. Bring to a boil, skim, cover and simmer gently for about an hour. If necessary, skim again. This makes a clear beef broth without seasonings.

For a more flavorful broth (1 quart), add a whole stalk of celery and leaves, 2 whole carrots, 1 potato, 2 tablespoons of tomato paste, or ½ cup of canned tomatoes or tomato juice. Add salt to taste. Cover, bring to a boil, lower heat, and simmer for about an hour. Add more water, if necessary. Remove the whole vegetables, place on a platter to cool, cut into small pieces, and return to broth. This gives a Beef Vegetable Soup with a real time saver built in. There should be enough for 2 good servings of Beef Vegetable Soup and about 2 cups of flavorful Beef Broth.

How to Freeze Beef Cuts

Once the steak is cut into smaller pieces, wrap each piece that you cannot use quickly, and store in the freezer. Use freezer paper to wrap each piece, squeezing the air out of the package by pressing it down with your hands to make it as compact as possible. Seal with freezer tape. Label with name of cut and date. These pieces are usually small and may get mislaid in the back of the freezer. To avoid this, take the separately wrapped cuts, place them together in a plastic bag, seal. The larger package is less likely to be mislaid.

If the cuts are placed in the refrigerator freezing compartment rather than in a regular freezer, use the meat within two weeks. If stored in a regular freezer at 0° F., use within two months for best quality and flavor.

When ready to use the meat, remove what is needed and thaw in the refrigerator rather than on a kitchen counter. Most people report that for best results, they place frozen meat in the refrigerator to thaw the night before it is to be used.

Note about knives: No special, expensive knife is needed for cutting up beef, or other meats. Any sharp knife a person has that is comfortable in the hand may be used. The knife must be very sharp and the person must feel secure about using it. A knife used for cutting meat should not come in contact with other metal because this dulls the blade. Don't put the knife in the drawer with other kitchen or tableware. People tell us they have to hide this knife from others in the household so it will not be used for purposes that spoil its edge.

Make a protective shield for the meat-cutting knife at no expense by simply taking two pieces of heavy cardboard a little longer and slightly wider than the knife blade. Seal the edges with heavy tape, leaving one end open to slide in the knife blade. When using, take special care in removing the knife from the shield, since it is only paper.

A Money-Saving Chicken Cutting Plan

You must have noticed that whole chickens usually sell for less per pound than those that are quartered or sold in separate parts such as breasts, thighs, drumsticks, etc. You may also have noticed that when you buy chicken in parts,

The Feel-Better Kitchen • 155

the liver, gizzard, and heart are not included. This way of buying chicken not only costs more but you get less chicken meat than in a whole chicken sold with the extras like liver included. These extras can often make a nourishing protein main dish for one person for a whole extra meal.

From the meat man's point of view, he charges for more service when he cuts up a chicken, and he makes more profit. Turn this around in your favor by cutting up whole chickens yourself. The savings are from 8 cents to 10 cents per pound. Since whole fryers weigh from 2½ to 3 pounds, you will be saving at least 20 cents a chicken every time you cut one up yourself. There is also the bonus saving of the extra meal made with the liver, gizzard, and heart that come with the whole chicken. The least that a meat protein serving costs per person is around 50 cents. Add this to the 20 cents to 25 cents saved by cutting up, and you find you save a total of 70 cents to 75 cents every time you cut up a chicken yourself rather than buying chicken parts.

May we beg you in the name of good nutrition never to buy chicken wings separately at the store unless the price is so low it's practically a giveaway. Chicken wings are mostly bone, skin, and sinew, usually very poor food value for the money. They give little protein nourishment when compared with other chicken cuts.

How to Cut Up a Whole Chicken

1. Place chicken on cutting surface. Turn chicken on side. To remove wing, start cutting on the inside of wing just over the joint. Let what looks like a white line at joint be your guide for cutting. Cut down and around joint. Repeat on other wing. (Figure 1)

2. To cut out backbone, place tail end on cutting surface. Place knife on one side of backbone and cut from neck along side of backbone, through rib joints to tail end. Repeat on other side of backbone. (Figures 2 & 3)

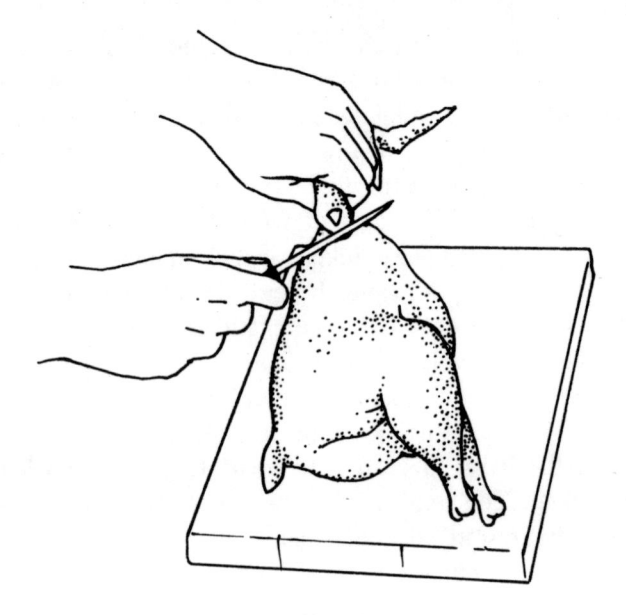

Figure 1

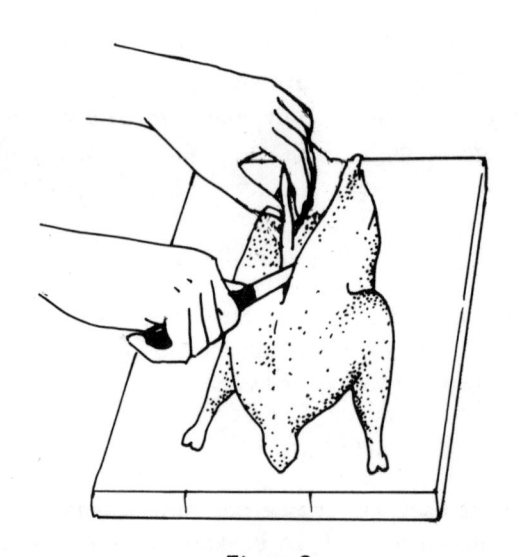

Figure 2

Figure 3

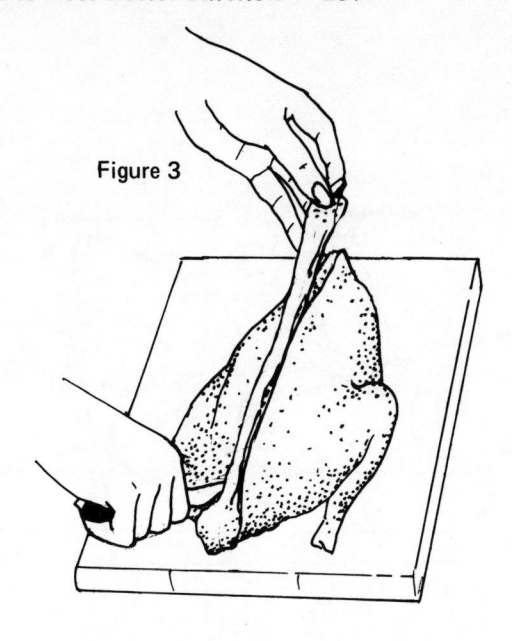

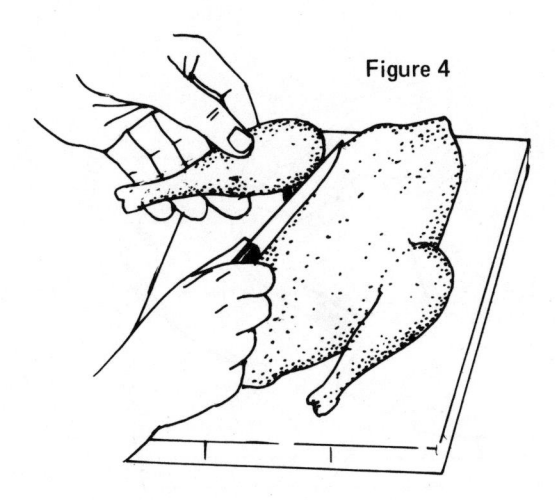

Figure 4

3. To cut legs, cut skin between thighs and body of chicken. Bend back leg until leg snaps loose. Then cut the leg from body of chicken. Repeat same on other leg. You can separate drumstick from thigh by cutting through joint. (Figures 4 & 5)

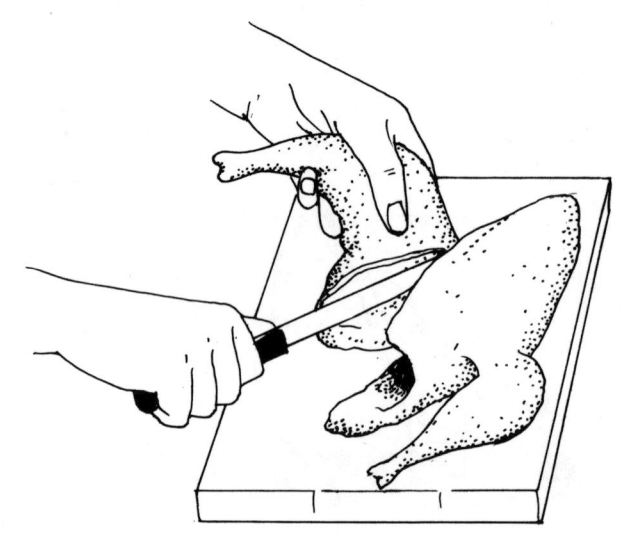

Figure 5

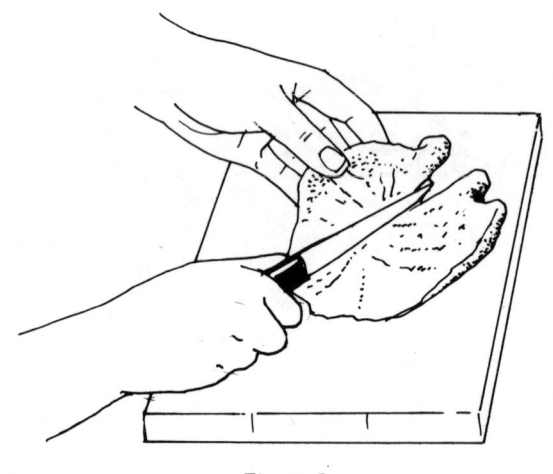

Figure 6

4. To cut breast in half, place breast skin side down on cutting board. Cut through to white spoon-shaped cartilage at the V of the neck. (Figure 6)

The Feel-Better Kitchen • 159

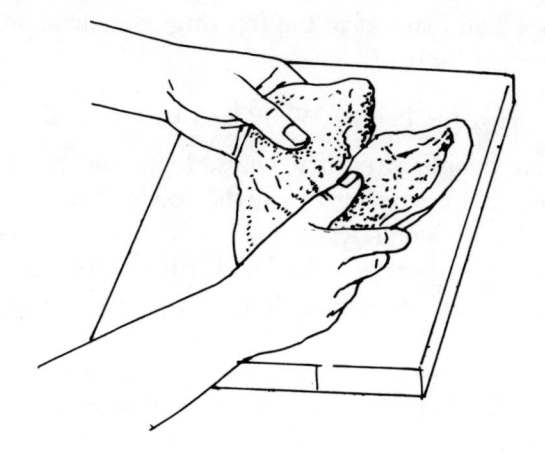

Figure 7

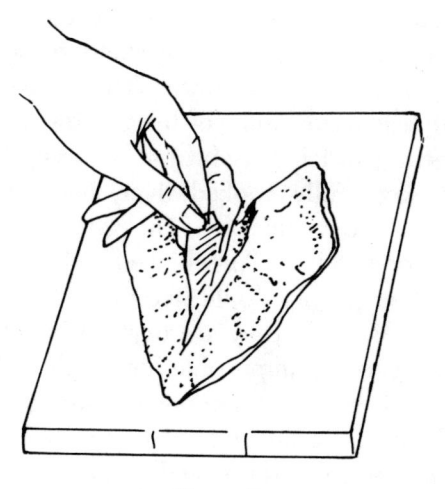

Figure 8

5. Hold breast firmly with both hands and bend back both sides. Push up with fingers to snap out the breastbone. This can be easily pulled out. Cut breast in half lengthwise. (Figures 7 & 8)

Any chicken pieces not to be used quickly should be wrapped and stored in the freezing compartment or freezer, as directed for beef.

Tips for People Who Can't Chew Well

Some people after fifty, whose teeth and gums are in poor shape, give up trying to eat the foods that they know they need. Many people who have trouble chewing end up eating plain hamburgers or meat loaf for the rest of their lives, and they eat only vegetables that are soft and mushy and tasteless.

Most people already have more than enough equipment in their kitchens for preparing food that is easy to chew and that will bring real variety to meals. For those who may not have them, we suggest two pieces of equipment. A meat grinder is a must. The old-fashioned, hand-operated kind will do very well, but if one already has the electrical kind, that is fine, too. The other piece of equipment is an old-fashioned grater. It can be the standard square type made of metal, or a simple flat grater. These two pieces of equipment properly used can be of the greatest help.

The meat grinder is useful for chopping beef, veal, lamb, pork, chicken, fully cooked liver, heart and kidney, and some fruits and vegetables. The grinder breaks down big pieces of food to little "prechewed" pieces, so to speak.

Many older people would like to eat food like raw carrots and raisins. Because they are dry, raisins often cut into the gums. Raw carrot is impossible for people who have difficulty chewing. Put the carrot and raisins through the food grinder, and both the taste and feel of these foods can be enjoyed. For a salad, simply add a small amount of mayonnaise or a favorite fruit dressing.

People who enjoy bread pudding often like the added touch of nuts and dried fruits but these do not soften enough during cooking for easy chewing. Grind such fruit as dried apricots or raisins along with the nuts, and they can be added to the pudding and chewed easily.

Properly cooked collard greens are also hard to chew. Grind the raw greens, cook in a small amount of water, and they can be enjoyed even by those with chewing problems.

The grinder is useful, too, to chop foods if a person has arthritic or rheumatic hands that make chopping no longer possible. Foods like celery, carrots, and certain firm greens can be chopped by putting them through the food grinder.

When grinding any meat, use the coarse blade of the grinder rather than the fine blade because the coarse blade leaves more texture in the meat. Most butchers will not grind meats other than beef, unless the customer comes to the store at a special hour. In fact, some butchers will not do this at all. Having one's own meat grinder does away with this problem, and allows for a wider choice of foods. For example, by grinding raw chicken, a delicious chicken loaf can be made as a change from the usual meat loaf. Or one can make interesting chicken balls instead of meatballs, or stuffed green peppers with chicken, or chicken-fried rice, or ground chicken can be mixed with cheese or eggs, or made into good chicken sandwich spreads.

A person with chewing problems need not always use a food grinder to prepare meals. Dishes made with milk and cheese can be a very nourishing change for people with chewing troubles. For example, easy-to-chew main dishes made with cheese include macaroni and cheese, Welsh rarebit on small cubes of toast, cheese soufflé, cheese and vegetable omelet, and a baked cheese strata of layered bread and cheese sauced with an egg-and-milk mixture.

Good Food Storage Makes Sense

Many people do not know enough about storing foods promptly and correctly. The result is they often have stomach pain, diarrhea, and mild food poisoning. "Something I ate didn't agree with me," may be more truly stated: "Something I ate stood out too long in the room and now it's causing me problems."

A household where the medicine chest is full of digestive remedies is often a telltale sign that the people living there are not following the rules of good food storage.

People who try these very simple rules may find a remarkable improvement in well-being and be able to save the expense and nuisance of using digestive remedies.

Over-All Safety Rules

1. Serve foods soon after cooking. Never let them stand long at room temperature. Refrigerate any leftover food promptly.
2. Keep hot foods hot (above 140° F.) and cold foods cold (below 40° F.).
3. Food may not be safe to eat if allowed to stand for more than 1 or 2 hours at temperatures between 60° and 120° F. This is the danger zone where food bacteria grow fast. Remember that the 1- to 2-hour limit includes the time taken for preparation of the food such as cutting up, chopping, washing, serving, etc.; and any time that the food is left out after serving. You can see that this allows for very little time for cooked food to stand around.

Common sense is a great help for safe food storage. In very hot weather, or in a very hot room, cut down "standing-out time" to as short a period as possible.

The cooling of large quantities of food can be hurried up by refrigerating in containers that are not deep, allowing more surface for quick cooling. It is advisable to refrigerate hot foods promptly, just so they are not so hot that they raise the refrigerator temperature above 45° F. Some people feel that this makes bigger utility bills but a better way to look at it is that this kind of storage avoids food spoilage and may well save a doctor's bill or even a trip to the hospital. It's a fact that foods that become spoiled through bacteria growth often do not change in appearance or in taste and have no bad smell. There is no warning that they may cause food poisoning or other distress.

Be Particularly Careful about These Foods

Whenever flour or other thickener is combined with fat and liquid as in the making of gravies and sauces, a seedbed for bacteria is present which, when the foods are allowed to stand at warm temperatures, can develop dangerously and causes digestive upsets and food poisoning. People should be very prompt in storing gravies, sauces, and certain puddings.

Other foods that can cause trouble unless refrigerated promptly are dishes made with eggs, such as cream pies, custard pies, or fillings made with custard, and meringue pies. Cakes, éclairs, and cream puffs with custard fillings require very prompt refrigeration and are not good choices for taking on picnics or for other occasions where they will stand out of the refrigerator for any length of time. Other foods especially likely to spoil are salads and sandwiches made with salad dressings containing eggs or milk products and little vinegar or other acids.

Bread stuffing for poultry and meats is such a dangerous medium for growth of bacteria that it deserves very special attention. If stuffing is made in advance, never fill a poultry or meat cavity with the stuffing and keep it in the refrigerator for some time before cooking. This can start severe bacteria contamination or production of toxins. Instead, make up stuffing, refrigerate it separately, and stuff the poultry or meat immediately before cooking. Again, when the cooked stuffed poultry or meat has been served, immediately remove the stuffing from the poultry or meat, and store in a separate container in the refrigerator.

Have you ever been to a Thanksgiving dinner where stuffed turkey was served and the turkey was left standing for hours on the table until a later meal when everyone helped themselves to cold turkey and stuffing? The next day, people say: "I have a stomach ache and nausea from eating too much," but the real reason for the upset is that the food produced toxins from standing at room temperature for a long period, and mild food poisoning occurred.

Cutting Boards Can Cause Trouble

Any place where raw meat, poultry, or fish is prepared, such as a counter top, table, or cutting board can become a dangerous source of food poisoning. Bacteria can work into tiny cracks or pores in boards or counters and contaminate the hands with bacteria or toxins that may get into the mouth, or they can contaminate foods such as salad greens, bread, etc., that are prepared in the same place. Many people have suffered painful infections in this way.

The way to avoid this is to scrub thoroughly any cutting or food preparation surface with hot soapy water and for good measure add some chlorine laundry bleach in the amount directed on the package.

Cutting knives for meat, fish, poultry should be treated as above with utmost care. They can contaminate other foods if not thoroughly cleaned after each use. Meat grinders, blenders, and can openers can also cause trouble unless completely cleaned after each use.

Hands and Food Spoilage

People can be very conscientious about keeping food preparation surfaces clean and still have trouble because they do not know that hands can spread bacteria and cause a serious upset in the system. If a person has just been handling raw meat, poultry, or fish and then handles salad greens or other food to be served raw without first washing hands with soap thoroughly, the food can be contaminated with bacteria and cause nausea and other symptoms of food poisoning. Thorough cooking destroys the bacteria but not everything is served cooked.

Safe Times for Storing Meats, Poultry, Fish

These foods should be stored in the meat compartment or coldest part of the refrigerator:

Chops, cutlets, roasts, and steaks keep safely in the refrigerator 3 to 5 days. To store in refrigerator, wrap them loosely, since partial drying of the surface aids keeping quality. Stored in the freezer at 0° F., these meats keep about 4 months.

Ground beef, stew meat, or variety meats are highly perishable: maximum storage time in the refrigerator is 1 to 2 days; in a freezer at 0° F, about 2 months.

Cooked meat, meat dishes, and gravy or meat broth can be stored for 1 to 2 days in refrigerator, and about 2 months in the freezer at 0° F.

Fresh chicken, loosely wrapped, or cooked chicken can be kept in the refrigerator for one to two days. In the freezer, at 0° F. an uncooked whole chicken will keep nine months; a whole cooked chicken, three.

Fish, shucked clams, oysters, shrimp, and scallops are best used the same day purchased; store in refrigerator.

Clams or lobster tails in shell can be stored in the refrigerator 2 days; in the freezer, 0° F., about 3 months.

Meats stored in freezer should be wrapped in moisture-proof material such as freezer paper, sealed, labeled, and dated.

Special Care with Frozen Meats, Poultry, Fish

Always thaw these foods in the refrigerator, not on a counter or table top at room temperature. These foods can be cooked without thawing but special care must be taken. Undercooked foods may not be safe to eat. Allow at least 1½ times as long to cook these foods frozen as they call for when thawed before cooking.

Check Refrigerator Temperature

Food keeps best in the refrigerator when the temperature is between 35° F. and 40° F. Foods spoil faster when the temperature is above 45° F.

Check the temperature in the refrigerator with an outdoor thermometer or a refrigerator thermometer. If necessary, adjust the temperature control, usually located inside the refrigerator.

Salt Sense

The feel-better eater is careful about salt. According to a leading nutritionist, the average consumer in this country takes in as much as ten times the amount of salt needed by the body. Like other foods, salt is needed to function but abuse in the use of salt causes problems.

For instance, salt is half sodium and half chloride. Those who suffer from hypertension know that a low sodium diet is important in its treatment. Recent studies have shown good but not conclusive evidence that a diet habitually high in salt may predispose susceptible individuals to hypertension.

As a safeguard, feel-better meals should avoid highly salted commercial convenience foods. Write the manufacturer about the salt content of a product if it is not given on the label. As a further common-sense move, use smaller amounts of iodized salt in cooking, and take the salt shaker from the table altogether.

In hot weather, there is greatly increased sweating, and then a little extra salt should be used.

It's important to realize that some foods are sodium-rich in themselves without added salt. These include fresh meats, fish, certain cheeses, poultry, eggs, and milk. Plant foods are usually low in sodium. Foods such as ham, bacon, salted butter and margarine, salted fish, olives, bread, and crackers have a high sodium content because of the salt used in processing. Most convenience foods such as cake mixes, canned vegetables, potato chips, etc., contain salt.

Besides food and table salt, drinking water may be a source of dietary sodium. Persons on sodium-restricted diets should check with the doctor or town health officials concerning the sodium content of the local water.

Canned Goods Cupboard

For some people, like Old Mother Hubbard, the canned goods cupboard is bare, and that's okay, if a person prefers it that way. For others who live in remote areas, or are storm-bound in long winters, canned goods are indispensable. They are convenient foods in compact form that store in small space, and when they are properly stored for a few months, there is very little nutrition loss.

Canned foods combine well with fresh or frozen foods to help provide variety and good nutrition. The fact that canned foods do not require refrigeration when stored unopened is a double blessing. A person who does not have a refrigerator can use these foods safely, and there are no utility charges for storing them.

It's good buying sense to take advantage of canned foods when vegetables or fruits are out of season or selling at high prices.

It's smart to keep an emergency shelf of canned foods for the times when a person cannot get out, is unwell, or pressed for time in preparing for a meal. Stock this shelf with nutritious foods like canned tuna, sardines, green leafy vegetables such as spinach, kale, mixed greens, etc., canned peas, carrots, canned tomatoes, canned sweet potatoes, canned milk, canned lima, kidney and other beans, canned fruits packed in water or light syrup, and canned juices.

Use Canned Liquids

The liquid in canned vegetables and fruits usually makes up one-third of the contents in the container. Since the water-soluble vitamins in canned foods are about equally distributed in the solids and liquids, you may be throwing away a considerable amount of these nutrients, for which money was paid, if the liquid is not used. Use the liquid from canned vegetables in soups, sauces, gravies, or in other ways, such as adding them to a vegetable cocktail drink. Canned vegetable liquids can be frozen for later use.

The same applies to canned fruits and their liquids. They contain important nutrients, too. Use the juice to sweeten lemonade or a fruit juice punch, or as part of the liquid in making gelatine desserts, or to sweeten cereals in place of sugar. This gives full benefit from the nutrients in the liquid and also gives more food for the money.

Good Storage Saves Nutrients

Canned goods should be stored in a cool, dry place for a limited time for best flavor and amount of nutrients retained. Nutrient loss can occur when storage temperature is high. In a study, canned fruits and vegetables stored at 65° F. for a year suffered 10 percent vitamin C loss. The same type of canned foods stored at 80° F. for a year resulted in a loss as high as 25 percent. Losses of other vitamins vary in canned fruits and vegetables according to how stable the vitamins are to heat. For example, some thiamine is lost when canned meats are stored. Canned pork lunch meat may lose approximately 20 percent of its thiamine in three months' storage, and up to 30 percent in six months when it is stored at 70° F.

Avoid storing canned foods at freezing temperature. This may cause glass containers to break or damage can seams. When opened, unused canned food should be stored, covered, in the refrigerator. To avoid a metallic taste, transfer food to another container with a tight cover.

The reaction of acid and sulfur in foods may cause the inside of the can to discolor. Neither this change nor any metallic taste developing on standing is harmful.

Canny Cupboard Tip

Many live-alone people buy only the little, individual pack cans in 8-ounce sizes. This is undoubtedly convenient, but the smaller packs usually cost more per ounce of food than the larger size cans. The manufacturer who packs food in 8-ounce cans has about the same labor costs and pays almost as much for a small container as a big one. He has to "tool up" differently to pack small cans and this costs him money, too. Fewer people buy small pack cans than those who buy the larger sizes. All these factors contribute to small size cans costing more per ounce of food than larger cans. But you can avoid this extra expense. How? Just buy food in 1-pound cans. Serve some at one meal. Store the unused portion tightly covered in the refrigerator, and use within a few days. This saves a lot of money.

14
The Feel-Better Shopper

OUR EXPERIENCE WITH FOOD SHOPPERS over fifty has shown that they have very serious problems. Many have been used to shopping for four to six people all their lives. As the children leave, the household shrinks to one or two people, and the remaining after-fifty person can't adjust to planning meals and shopping on that scale. Some don't recognize the problem. They continue shopping as they always did. Then they find they are throwing away so much food, and both food and money are wasted. It is very discouraging. We found that many people become so frustrated with this situation, they turn off on shopping for balanced meals altogether. They live on TV dinners, packaged or canned foods, and junk snacks and beverages. This is a tragedy. It is responsible for the poor health and low spirits of many older people.

To help solve this problem, we made a basic weekly shopping checklist for people to tape to a cupboard or refrigerator door. This covers all the basic foods needed in daily meals in amounts for one person. In this way, the after-fifty person making up a shopping list won't skip any important food in the feel-better plan.

The Feel-Better Shopper • 171

There's a great advantage, too, in keeping a shopping list "loose" or "open" rather than tightly closed. If the list is too detailed, the shopper may miss a lot of bargains in the store. When the list, for instance, covers seven servings of vitamin A-rich foods (and you are now well aware what they are), you can quickly shift from frozen spinach to frozen turnip greens in the store if the turnip greens are cheaper.

Here's the checklist to refer to when making up a weekly shopping list. Soon you'll just do it naturally, and can pass the checklist on to a friend.

Basic Weekly Checklist for Feel-Better Foods

	Servings per Week	Amount per Serving
Red meat	2 to 3	3 to 4 ounces, uncooked (no bones or fat)
Chicken	2 to 3	3 to 4 ounces, uncooked (no bones or fat)
Fish	1 to 2	3 to 4 ounces, uncooked (no bones)
Eggs	3 to 5	
Cheese	2 to 4	1 ounce
Dried beans	1 to 2	½ cup, cooked
Vitamin A rich foods	7	½ cup, cooked
Vitamin C rich foods	7	½ cup juice or 1 medium piece fruit
Salad fixings	7 to 14	½ to 1 cup
Other fruits and vegetables	7 to 14	½ cup, cooked, or 1 medium piece fruit
Milk	14	1 cup
Whole grain bread and/or breakfast cereals	14	1 slice of bread, 1 ounce of dry cereal, or ½ to ¾ cup of cooked cereal
Other bread and cereal foods such as macaroni, noodles, grits, rice, spaghetti, cornmeal	14	½ to ¾ cup cooked

You will want to add to that list each week whatever staples you need to replace. Here's a brief checklist:

Staples Checklist

Margarine
Butter
Peanut Butter
Oil
Other fat
Tea
Coffee
Sugar or other sweetener
Salt
Pepper
Spices and herbs
Packaged puddings
Vinegar
Jam or jelly
Mustard
Ice cream

Our feel-better friends found it was wiser to make up a shopping list only after checking first the cupboard, refrigerator, and freezer to be sure they didn't already have the protein makings of a main dish in the house. They also checked on leftover fruits and vegetables and could often cross off one or two servings from the shopping list for the week to come. Taped lists of contents on the refrigerator and freezer are handy for this checking.

Even with less than a whole serving of cooked chicken or meat in the refrigerator, a nice main dish can be made, as we have already discovered. Chicken and noodles is a good example. And there's one less main dish to shop for, and a dollar or more saved.

Our experience shows that even with the cost of food outrageously high, food expenses came down when people learned to shop better, store food better, and avoid waste by such checking at home.

The Feel-Better Shopper • 173

Try the Buddy Shopping System

Because of the way most foods are sold, it's hard to buy protein foods such as meat and chicken in the small amounts required for one person. One easy solution is to follow the cut-your-own-meat plan of buying beef and chicken. If this plan is not followed, chicken can be bought by the part desired, and meat is available in small pieces, but this always costs more, often much more. There is a better way.

Find a shopping buddy with similar tastes in food. Then two friends can buy a whole chicken and split it in half at home for each to share. They'll save money and avoid monotony in their meals.

The buddy system is a great way to save not only when buying chicken, but also for many other foods that are sold in amounts too large for one person to use up, a whole melon, for example. Two people, each living alone, can buy in larger quantities at considerable savings, items such as cooking or salad oil, margarine, flour, cereals, spices, nonfat dry milk in packets, potatoes, onions—any food that is cheaper in larger packages and can be divided conveniently at home.

Shopping buddies sometimes make up trios and even quartets who shop together for certain items that are much cheaper in large sizes, or are featured at a sale price for a large quantity. When the food is unpacked at home, each buddy brings his or her own container to take home a share of the bargain buy.

Shopping buddies can have fun together at the store. They can apply feel-better ideas and tricks to save a lot of money, helping each other to spot the very best buys. Two heads are better than one and combining shopping savvy and experience should bring better savings and better food for each buddy.

It was our experience that shopping buddies often became such good friends that they began making meals for each other. This brought them much more variety in their food, more enjoyment eating together than alone, and more richness in their lives.

Giving Up Some Bad Shopping Habits

The Feel-Better Group included shoppers with years of experience and they had many good ideas to share. However, when one of the group suggested, "Always look for the advertised specials in the newspaper and put them on your shopping list," Mrs. Shell replied: "No way!" There was a shocked silence and Mrs. Shell had a lot of convincing to do.

She explained that if you automatically put advertised specials on your shopping list, it may block you from much better buys that you could find when you get to the store. For example, recently a supermarket featured as a special a beef cut with tenderloin removed for $1.49 a pound. After checking the meat counter as well as other sections of the store, the following proved to be better choices for the money that day: beef liver was selling at the regular price of 89 cents a pound; chuck steak was selling for 69 cents a pound; cottage cheese, a good protein food, was selling for 98 cents a pound, and eggs, another fine protein food, for 63 cents a dozen. If a person had bought the $1.49 beef special without checking prices of other good protein foods in the store the same day, they would have paid 80 cents more a pound for the beef special than for the chuck steak selling at the regular price. Both cuts give the same amount of lean meat. The meat has the same good complete protein, so the nutritional value is identical. Why not get more for the money with a little careful checking?

We have found this problem with so-called specials to be true also with canned goods, fresh produce, dairy products, and many other foods. If, for instance, canned corn is an advertised special, always check the other brands on the shelf before buying. Often, the advertised special is set up in a large special display, away from other brands of the same product. Always go to the shelf where this product is sold, check if it is really cheaper than other brands of similar quality, and only then make your decision to buy. We have saved many, many dollars this way, and so have our friends, now that they are on to this little piece of shopping strategy.

Certainly, make note of specials when a store advertises them. But look and compare before you buy.

A Careful Look at Coupons

Mrs. Shell spoiled a lot of people's fun when she said that shopping coupons are one of the costliest games a shopper can play. But don't go away. We have a replacement for that game that will be just as much fun and save more money.

Studies show that 80 percent of shoppers use coupons. But that doesn't make them smart shoppers. It may be quite the contrary. Like the advertised specials, the couponed foods should only be bought when they are truly a best buy for you, and after making careful comparisons at the store. Coupons often induce people to buy foods for which they have no need. That's waste, and it makes food bills higher.

Coupons are used by food merchandisers for several reasons, most of them not to your advantage. The first is basic. It's to get you into the supermarket. Once you're in, the merchants know you are going to spend money. Coupons are also used to get you to try new products. These are often elaborately packaged, and thus high in price. They are sometimes a fancy form of a good basic food. It may be available elsewhere in the store at much less cost. Check it. Oddly enough, the plainer version of the food is often more nutritious.

Another reason for couponing is when a manufacturer wants to overcome the successful competition of another company making the same type of product. He offers a coupon to get you to come back to his brand. Because he is so anxious to get your business, this may be a worthwhile coupon, a real saving, but check first at the store. Couponing is also done when manufacturers and stores do not move products fast enough and there is a pile-up at the warehouse. The coupon is planned to overcome sales lag. Sometimes, if the product is a feel-better food, coupons can bring very good buys, but check before buying.

A popular form of supermarket ad offers a saving of an over-all sum such as $1.75 if all its weekly coupons are used by the customer. But what are the coupons buying? Are they feel-better foods? Or are they gimmicky foods? Worthless snacks? Or heavily processed foods that do not offer the most nutrition for the money? You know how to tell the difference. When in doubt, read ingredient listings and nutrition panels on the label. You'll soon know if the coupon is worth using.

And what is our replacement for the coupon game? Get yourself a little notebook that can be carried in a woman's purse or a man's pocket. Collect all the coupons you like. Take them to the store. Apply the standards for judging a good coupon buy. If you find it's worthwhile, note what you saved, using the coupon, in your little book. If you find it's not a best buy, note the amount you saved by *not* buying it, and discard the coupon. You'll be amazed at how high the figures mount in that little book. This is a coupon game that you can win every time!

Shopping Savers—Avoiding Tricks and Traps

After you've overcome the peril of making too tight a list for shopping, and resisted unthinking use of advertised specials and coupons, you're about ready for the adventure of the supermarket. Here there is great good as well as the bad and the indifferent. Just as a person who can't read can't do very much for himself in the world today, a person who doesn't know the art of reading and figuring out food labels is also at a great disadvantage. First, the story; then we'll go on to other things you can do in the supermarket to bring home better food for much less money.

The Art of Label Reading

Labels on packages and cans are like road signs that help you get to where you want to go, if you follow them carefully. Labels give the weight of the foods in the container, the number of servings, and the style of food such as cream style or whole kernel corn, or whether a fruit is packed in light or heavy syrup, or in its own juice.

Two very vital helps toward better food shopping are the ingredient listing on labels, and the nutrition information panels, where provided. It is important to know how to use these aids. They can provide an excellent education for everyone who shops.

Ingredient Listings

Ingredient listings can help you to decide whether the food inside the container is a good one to include in feel-better meals. When an ingredient listing is given, it's a cue to many things. The most important thing to know is that by law the ingredients are listed according to the quantity in which they are included in the product. The ingredient in the largest amount is listed first. For instance, let's make up an ingredient listing like this: tomato sauce, spaghetti, meatballs, flavoring, etc. The experienced label reader would know at once that there was more sauce in the product than spaghetti, and more spaghetti than meatballs. This is a very good way to check how much food and nutrition your money is buying.

Now let's try reading an actual label for a ready-to-eat cereal to see what it can tell us:

Ready-Sweetened, Ready-to-Eat Cereal

Sugar, corn, wheat and oat flour, hydrogenated vegetable oil, salt, artificial coloring, sodium ascorbate (C), vitamin A palmitate, niacinamide, ascorbic acid (C), zinc oxide, iron, natural orange, lemon, cherry and other natural flavorings, thiamin hydrochloride (B_1), pyridoxine hydrochloride (B_6), riboflavin (B_2), folic acid and vitamin D_2, preservatives BHA and BHT

You can see that this means that there is more sugar in this cereal than any other ingredient listed, and there is less actual cereal—corn, wheat and oat flour, than sugar! We in the Feel-Better Group decided that we would not buy or use any product in which sugar was the first item in the ingredient listing. Some people decided that they didn't want the product if sugar was the second item listed either.

Let's try reading another label:

Vitamin C Enriched Canned Fruit Drink (not juice), 46 fluid ounces or 1 quart, 14 ounces

Water, sugar and corn sweeteners, concentrated orange juice, concentrated lemon juice, natural flavors, fumaric and citrus acids (provide tartness), vitamin C, artificial colors; contains 10 percent fruit juices

As you see, the item in largest amount in this product is water! Next comes sugar and sweeteners in an amount larger than the fruit juices. You can tell there is not enough of these juices present to provide much vitamin C because the listing includes added vitamin C and the label states "enriched with vitamin C." But the real booby-trap is the statement on the label: "Contains 10 percent fruit juices." In other words, you might as well say that in a 46 ounce can of this product, only 4.6 ounces are juices. After studying labels like these, the Feel-Better Group decided not to buy any product in which the first item listed as an ingredient was water.

Ingredient listings will also tip you off to the use of artificial flavoring and artificial color in foods, and to chemical preservatives and other additives. Use ingredient listings wisely in the store and they will help to locate the feel-better foods at the supermarket.

Nutrition Labeling

You already know how to get the nutrition you need daily to feel your best. The Handy Food Finder, chapter 7, and the Daily Food Guide, page 79, can be used for reference. In addition, the nutritional panels on labels in the store are another good way to help choose foods that fit your nutritional needs. These panels do not appear on all labels but many products now carry them. They are required by law only when the manufacturer makes any claim about the nutritive value of the product, puts on the package nutritional information of any kind, or adds nutrients to fortify a food. When the nutrition information panel is used, it must show:

- *Serving size* (A portion such as one slice, one cup, or 3 ounces)
- *Servings per package or container*
- *The percent of the U. S. Recommended Daily Allowance* for protein, vitamin A, vitamin C, thiamine, riboflavin, niacin, calcium, and iron furnished by a serving of the food as it comes from the package

The percentages of the USRDA are given in increments of 2 percent (2, 4, 6, 8) up to 10 percent; of 5 percent (10, 15, 20, etc.) up to 50 percent; and 10 percent (50, 60, 70, etc.) above 50 percent. Important: an asterisk (*) means that the food provides none, or less than 2 percent of the USRDA for that nutrient. In addition, the nutrition panel may show the following:

- The percentage of USRDA for any of 12 additional vitamins and minerals furnished by a serving
- The percentage of calories that comes from fat and the amount of polyunsaturated fat, saturated fat, and cholesterol furnished by a serving of the specified size

This helps persons who have been advised by a doctor to limit amount of fat and cholesterol in the diet.

- The amount of sodium furnished by a serving of food

This is important to persons who have been advised by a doctor to limit amount of salt in the diet. This is particularly helpful when buying convenience foods as they tend to be higher in salt content.

- Nutrition information for a serving of the food cooked or prepared in combination with other foods according to directions given on the label

Special Note for After-Fifty People

The U.S. Recommended Dietary Allowances are based on the amount of nutrients needed for all sex-age groups. This is sometimes more than is needed by many people. For persons after fifty, the percentages for several nutrients are less than the USRDA. The following percentages of the USRDA are recommended for these men and women by the U.S. Department of Agriculture:

Allowances for Food Energy and Percentages of the U.S. Recommended Daily Allowances Needed to Meet the Recommended Dietary Allowances for Men and Women Whose Age is 51 Plus

	Food Energy Calories	Protein	Vitamin A	Vitamin C	Thiamine	Riboflavin	Niacin	Calcium	Iron
		Percent of U.S. Recommended Daily Allowance
Male	2,400	90	100	75	80	90	35	80	60
Female	1,800	75	80	75	70	65	25	80	60

By studying this table, it will be seen that after-fifty people in many cases can plan their meals around less than the USRDA percentages. It would be a waste of money to buy food according to the full 100 percent allowances in most cases. However, our Food Finder, chapter 7, has been adjusted to give the special percentage figures recommended for people after fifty. Use the Finder to avoid complicated calculating at the store when reading nutrition panels. Mrs. Shell has done all the work for you.

Compare Price by Weight or Measure

Comparison often helps people to make the best choice for the money among different size packages or brands of the same food. In states where unit pricing has been legislated, this work is done for the customer. Otherwise, they have to do it themselves, but it isn't very hard and it can save a lot of money. Just take the total number of ounces, pounds, quarts, etc., on the package, divide this figure into the price, and you have the price per unit. Do the same for other packages or brands of the same food. Compare the price per unit, such as an ounce of the other packaged foods, and you will soon determine the best buy for the money. This is important because often packages, boxes, bottles will look larger than others to the eye, but when actual weights are compared, this is found to be an illusion. Experiment with this at the supermarket, and you will soon catch on to the trick of figuring out the most for the money.

We do want to stress that price alone should never be the deciding factor when buying food. Quality is important for good nutrition, eating pleasure, and for avoiding waste. A food may be cheaper but if it isn't good quality, it will probably be thrown away and the money is wasted.

Why Pay a Convenience Tax?

We call it a convenience tax when you pay considerably more for a product because the manufacturer has given you a service such as cooking, or put several ingredients together in one package that you could easily do yourself for much less money. True, you might spend a little more time. If you'd rather have the money, it's easy to vote no on the convenience tax.

Here are some examples of these products.

Sauce and seasoning mix packets. Recently at the store, a cheese sauce mix in a 1¼ ounce plastic-coated package cost 39 cents. The ingredients listed were Cheddar cheese, corn starch, whey solids, salt, soybean oil, bleu cheese, Romano cheese, buttermilk solids, paprika, turmeric and spice. At 39 cents a package, the cost of those ingredients per pound would be $4.99! You also have to add your own milk, at extra cost. That's a very high convenience tax. A tasty cheese sauce can be made at home very simply by adding a quarter-cup of any grated cheese to three quarters of a cup of homemade white sauce, and seasoning to taste. Then, too, some of us like the taste better when a sauce is made with fresh ingredients.

In a seasoning mix packet for Sloppy Joes priced at 29 cents for 1½ ounces, the ingredients were onion, sugar, salt, flour, precooked and dried potato with sodium sulfite (a preservative), spices, and garlic. The cost per pound for those ingredients at the packet price would be $3.09. The directions suggest using a pound of ground beef, a can of tomato paste, and the seasoning mix. In other words, for a bit of flavoring, you are adding 29 cents to the cost of making a relatively economical dish. A little chopped onion, salt, herb of your choice such as thyme or oregano, a bit of garlic, and some leftover cooked vegetables could give the same result for less—and without additives.

Seasoned coating mixes for breading chicken or other meats carry a high convenience tax. The day we bought a 4¾-ounce package containing two packets of coating mix, it cost 87 cents. If you use this product, try this experiment. Empty out one of the little packets into a measuring cup, instead of into a bag as suggested. You'll find it measures only a half-cup. For that you pay anywhere from 40 cents to 46 cents. If you are willing to spend a little time to avoid paying a convenience tax that is very high indeed, measure into a bag a quarter-cup of flour, a quarter-cup dry bread crumbs, ⅛ teaspoon paprika, salt and pepper to taste, and a sprinkling of garlic salt, if desired. Use a quarter-cup of vegetable oil or milk to coat the chicken lightly and shake off excess liquid. Place two or three pieces of chicken in the bag with the coating mixture, and shake until evenly coated. Bake as you usually do. When Mrs. Shell figured out the cost of her own coating mix and the plastic bag, she found it only came to 12 cents. Is a convenience tax of 32 cents on one packet of this mix really worth paying?

Here are examples of high convenience tax products from the frozen foods department. On a recent shopping trip, frozen broccoli cuts in a 20-ounce bag were priced at 90 cents. A 10-ounce package of broccoli in cheese sauce sold for 71 cents, and the same size package of broccoli in butter sauce for 73 cents. Studying the weight of the package does not show how much of the package is broccoli and how much is sauce. So we have to look at it another way. Ten ounces of the plain broccoli cuts as priced above would come to 45 cents. If a butter sauce were added at home, it could not possibly cost the 26 cents difference in price between the plain frozen broccoli and the butter sauce pack. So 26 cents is being paid for sauce and service. With the broccoli in cheese sauce product, the difference comes to 28 cents.

Slice the cost of cheese. Sometimes the convenience tax is for a very small service, such as slicing cheese. In a supermarket cheese case, individually wrapped slices of American process cheese were selling at $1.39 for a 12-ounce package ($1.85 a pound). In the same case, natural mild Cheddar cheese was selling by the piece at $1.59 a pound. That's a saving of 26 cents, just for slicing a pound of cheese yourself. Since the American slices are made with cheese food, there is added moisture, and consequently less nutrition than in the natural Cheddar cheese. Careful shopping and trying different kinds of bulk cheeses will bring more flavor and variety in cheese for your table. These cheeses keep well when tightly wrapped at home and stored in the refrigerator.

A *dramatic drink example.* On a recent shopping trip, one of the most popular powdered instant orange breakfast drinks was selling for 85 cents for a 9-ounce jar, which makes 2 quarts. There was also a special on unsweetened frozen 100 percent orange concentrate that made three quarts for 59 cents. Following the suggestions on how to use frozen orange juice for live-alones by liquefying it a little at a time, the product was convenient to use, and it yielded an extra quart of orange juice compared with the powdered mix. The cost per quart for the frozen orange juice was 20 cents whereas the cost per quart for the drink mix was 43 cents. Another dramatic example of a high convenience tax.

Canned meat spreads. These products are very easy to use but the convenience comes very high. When a 3-ounce can of deviled luncheon meat spread sells for 39 cents, the cost per pound for this meat is $2.08. When deviled ham in a 4.5-ounce can sells for 67 cents a can, it's $2.38 a pound. Think how much a person could make with bits of leftover ham before it would come to $2.38 a pound! Besides, this product contains 32 percent fat. When deviled ham spread is made at home, all the visible fat is removed, so there is more meat and more protein nutrition for the money. Canned meat spreads have a high salt content. In fact, most convenience foods come with a high salt tax as well as a high convenience tax.

A recent newcomer to the supermarket shelves is canned meatballs without gravy. A 7-ounce can sells for $1.98. This means that a pound of these meatballs would cost $4.52. If this product is used by people over fifty who can't have gravy, and there are many of them, they are paying an enormous convenience tax for meat. Make meat balls without gravy at home and save dollars.

Cold Cuts and the Convenience Tax

We have already said that we don't feel that cold cuts bring the best protein nutrition for the money spent. How many realize how high the prices are on these meats? During a recent price check, a 6-ounce package of beef salami was 99 cents which comes to $2.64 a pound. A 4-ounce package of white meat chicken roll was 69 cents, or $2.76 a pound. An 8-ounce package of chicken bologna sold for $1.18; an 8-ounce package of tongue and blood loaf, 99 cents; a 4-ounce package of hard salami, 99 cents, or $3.96 a pound! You be the judge of how much fine protein food you could buy for $3.96. Some of our feel-better friends bought all the meat they needed for less than $4.00 a week, using fresh cuts of meat, chicken, or fish.

Avoiding Breakfast Cereal Traps

There are many traps in the breakfast cereal section of the supermarket, so proceed with care. Two of them are especially devastating. It didn't take our Feel-Better Group long to realize that one should never buy a breakfast cereal where the first item in the ingredient listing is sugar. The second thing they decided was that they would never buy breakfast cereals in individual small packs. Never seems a very rigid word. But let's look at why "never" is really the right word. One day in the supermarket, we found that a special variety pack of ten individual single serving boxes of ready-to-eat cereal was selling for 89 cents. When figured at cost per pound, this came to $1.56 a pound for ready-to-eat cereal. The same day there was a variety six pack of sugar-coated, ready-to-eat cereals that weighed 5 ounces and came to 63 cents. At the same store, an 8-ounce package of both cornflakes and wheat flakes cost only 45 cents each without the sugar coating.

The 10-pack unsweetened cereal came to 9 cents for a 1-ounce serving, not counting the milk that usually accompanies it. The sweetened individual packs came to 13 cents a 1-ounce serving, and the plain bulk package of cornflakes and wheat flakes came to 6 cents a serving, without milk. The reason that we mention milk is that the manufacturer gives nutrition information on the package with, and without, milk. As you know, the milk is necessary to improve the quality of the incomplete protein in the cereal, and to make it into a good breakfast dish.

The Either/Or Trap

Many consumer experts on TV and radio compare the cost of a small box of cereal with a large box, and that's a good way to begin such considerations. But this type of comparison alone can blind a person to the real cereal bargains that pay off nutritionally. The next time you go to the supermarket, to discover the way to get the most nutritious cereal for the money, take a look at the cereals that require a little cooking time. On the day that we did this, we found that a serving of oatmeal without milk came to only 3½ cents.

Whenever you see a comparison made that considers only either this or that product, keep looking. There may well be a better buy. We call this the either/or trap. Beyond either and or there's more, and this may be the best buy of all.

Big Isn't Necessarily Better

When you're strolling down the supermarket aisles, and you come upon a great big, big display of one type of product, beware! It may be wonderful food at good prices. Then again it may not. Be warned that big displays usually mean foods that bring high profits. That's why they give them so much space. These items may not have much nutritive value. One of the ironies of modern food merchandising is that in some cases the less value a food has for the body, the bigger the advertising drive put behind it, and the higher the amount of money spent to promote it. Soft drinks are the best example of this kind of marketing. Big advertising. Big displays. Big profit. Low or no food value.

Another tip. Don't shop the shelves only at eye level. That's often where the high profit items are. Look elsewhere, especially at floor level, in the hope of less expensive buys.

Best Fresh Fruit Buys

We have covered the selection and storage of fresh fruit in chapter 12, "The Feel-Better Kitchen: How to Plan for It." The over-all rule for best buys and best quality and flavor in fresh fruit is to buy fruits as they come into season. Here is a calendar of fresh fruits and their seasons to help you look for the best buys and the most enjoyment.

Fresh Fruit In Season

January	February	March
Grapefruit	Grapefruit	Grapefruit
Oranges	Oranges	Oranges
Tangelos		Pineapples
Tangerines		

April	May	
Grapefruit	Grapefruit	
Pineapple	Pineapple	
Strawberries	Strawberries	
	Watermelon	

June	July	August
Apricots	Apricots	Blueberries
Blueberries	Blueberries	Cantaloupe
Cantaloupe	Cantaloupe	Grapes
Cherries	Cherries	Honeydews
Honeydews	Grapes	Limes
Lemons	Lemons	Peaches
Limes	Limes	Pears
Peaches	Peaches	Plums
Plums and Prunes	Plums	Prunes
Strawberries	Prunes	Watermelon
Watermelons	Watermelon	

September	October	November
Grapes	Apples	Apples
Honeydews	Grapes	Tangelos
Peaches	Pears	Tangerines
Pears		
Plums		
Prunes		

December

Apples
Tangelos
Tangerines

This is a general guide, but factors such as size of crop, weather, shipping delays, disease, etc., will have a direct effect on availability and cost of fresh fruit.

Operation Alert!

For some people, food shopping is a big bore. But that need never be.

The supermarket is a great place for keeping alert and lively-minded. Food shopping is a battle of wits between the food sellers and the food buyers, and it's great fun to come out a winner. There are plenty of excellent, nourishing foods at the supermarket, and there are some that are not. Picking and choosing, comparing and deciding, will keep anyone on their toes when the job is well done.

Those who want to sharpen their shopping talents might like to do what we do. We often go to the supermarket not to shop but to watch people buy. This has taught us a great deal. Why don't you try it some day when you're feeling relaxed and have the time?

Watch the grabbers in the store rush up to shelves, grab anything they need without looking at weights, quality, or prices, and rush on to the next thoughtless buy. Grabbers are losers, you can bet on that.

The Feel-Better Shopper

Watch people pick out gimmicky packages with hardly any contents. Most of the manufacturer's money has gone into bright plastic and art design, and he can't afford to put much food inside the package.

Watch the folks who can never resist a cute little bottle, buy herbs and spices in glass for twice as much as those packed in paper boxes or in metal.

Listen to the tale of poor nutrition that some shopping carts tell—carts piled high with expensive instant foods, salty snacks, carbonated drinks, and no fresh fruit, milk, dark bread, or meat.

Watch the bee-line shoppers. They have a habit, when buying food, of always making a bee-line for the same section of the store instead of checking out different sections—frozen foods, dried foods, canned, and fresh—for the best buy.

Watch a shopper buy a 10-ounce package of frozen broccoli when there's a great big bunch on special the same day in the produce department—much more vegetable for less money.

Watch a shopper buy big fresh oranges, expensively priced out of season, when orange juice concentrate is selling at from 29 cents to 39 cents a 6-ounce can, an inexpensive source of vitamin C.

Watch people buy prepackaged coleslaw mix for as much as 98 cents a pound when fresh cabbage is selling for only 10 cents a pound.

Watch a shopper buy a bottle of olives, or a jar of pickled onions, or other doodads for the same price as a generous serving of fresh meat.

Food shopping is a fascinating game. Play it for all it's worth and enjoy it.

15
The Feel-Better Cookbook

THE MOST OFTEN heard reason for older people not eating well is: "I just can't seem to cook for one person."

Now they can. Here are one-serving recipes for delicious, feel-better food. Some recipes make two to three servings for such dishes as meat loaf or puddings that are welcome more than once in a week's meals. Others, such as Banana Bread, are planned for freezing by the slice to serve as desired.

One-Pot Chicken and Rice

Makes 1 serving

> 1 serving chicken, such as breast or leg
> 2 teaspoons of vegetable oil
> ¼ onion, chopped
> 3 tablespoons of raw rice
> 1 cup of hot water
> Salt and pepper to taste

Cook chicken in oil until golden brown, about 10 minutes on each side. Remove to plate.

Add onion and raw rice to fat in pan and cook over low heat until rice and onion are golden color, not brown.

Add browned chicken and water. Season to taste. Cover and bring to a boil. Stir. Cover, lower heat and simmer until chicken and rice are done, about 20 to 25 minutes.

Chicken in a Pot

Note. Use pan or pot with tightly fitting cover.

Makes 1 serving

1 cup of water
1 serving of chicken such as ½ breast or leg
1 medium potato, peeled and sliced or cubed
1 medium carrot, cleaned and cut into small pieces
1 small onion, sliced
Salt and pepper to taste

Pour water into medium size pot. Add chicken. Cover. Bring water to boil. Lower heat and gently simmer chicken for 25 minutes.

Add potato, carrot, onion, and seasonings. Cover. Continue to cook until vegetables are tender. To prevent sticking, add hot water, should it be needed.

Variations
1. Add 2 to 3 tablespoons of chopped parsley or celery leaves
2. Add ¼ cup of green beans, peas or lima beans
3. Add ¼ cup of tomatoes
4. Add herbs to your liking

Note. When you want chicken for a sandwich, cook 1½ servings. Save extra for sandwich filling.

Meat Loaf

Makes 3 to 4 servings

Note. Buy one pound of ground beef. Use ¼ pound for a hamburger or other ground-meat recipe. Use the rest to make meat loaf.

> ¾ pound of ground beef
> 1 cup of fresh white or whole wheat bread crumbs
> ¼ cup of tomato juice or tomato sauce or milk
> 1 medium-size egg
> 2 tablespoons of finely chopped onion
> Salt to taste

Preheat oven to 350° F. Put all the ingredients into a bowl. Mix well.

If mixture seems dry, add a small amount of liquid, a teaspoon at a time, mixing well before adding more liquid. If it seems too wet, add a small amount of bread crumbs.

Shape into a loaf and place in baking pan. Bake at 350° F., uncovered, about 50 to 60 minutes.

Variations. Meat loaf "flavor" can be changed by adding one of the following in amounts to suit your taste: curry powder, chili powder, chopped green pepper or celery, grated or cooked carrot or mixed vegetables, chopped parsley or grated cheese.

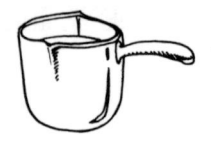

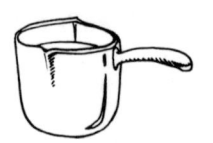

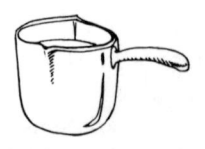

Double Duty Recipe For Meat Loaf and Meatballs
Shape half the meat loaf mixture into a loaf. Shape the remaining mixture into four to six meatballs, placing meat loaf and meatballs in the same pan so they do not touch each other. Bake at 350° F. for about 40 to 45 minutes.

Top-of-the-Stove Macaroni and Cheese Main Dish

Makes 1 serving

> 2 cups of water
> ¼ teaspoon of salt
> ⅓ to ½ cup of macaroni
> 2 tablespoons of milk or water or pan drippings
> 2 tablespoons of dry nonfat milk
> Dry mustard, to taste
> 2 ounces of cut-up or grated Cheddar-type cheese

Pour 2 cups water into small (1 quart) saucepan. Add salt. Bring to rolling boil. Add macaroni and cook until tender. Drain. Put macaroni in same pan used to cook it. In a cup, mix 2 tablespoons water, dry milk and dry mustard. Pour over cooked macaroni.

Using low heat, cook until milk is hot. Do not allow to boil. Gently stir in cheese and heat until cheese is melted, no longer.

May be served at once. If you like a thicker sauce, remove from heat, cover pan, and allow to stand 1 to 2 minutes. For a thinner sauce, add a teaspoon or more hot water.

Variations
1. In place of water and milk, use 3 tablespoons of yogurt or thick buttermilk
2. Add two stuffed green olives which have been sliced or chopped

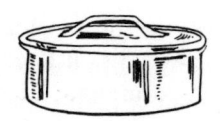

Spinach and Egg-Fry Main Dish

Makes 1 serving

> 1 egg
> 1 tablespoon of milk
> 1 tablespoon of finely grated cheese
> Salt and pepper to taste
> 2 teaspoons of margarine or oil
> ¾ cup of chopped raw spinach

Combine and beat egg, milk, grated cheese, salt, and pepper; set aside.

Melt and heat fat in fry pan. When hot, add and stir-fry spinach for about a minute.

Pour mixture over spinach in fry pan. Scramble and cook over low heat until eggs are set.

Pan-Fried Fish

Makes 1 serving

> ¼ to ⅓ pound of fish fillet (cod or flounder or perch or sole), cut into serving pieces
> 3 tablespoons of flour or cornmeal
> Salt and pepper to taste
> Sprinkling of paprika
> 3 teaspoons of oil or fat
> Lemon juice

Pat fish dry. Set aside. Mix flour or cornmeal with salt, pepper and paprika. Dip fish in flour mixture, coating it evenly.

Heat two teaspoons oil or fat in medium size fry pan. Fry fish about 5 to 6 minutes, or until golden brown on one side. Using a wide turner, gently lift fish and add 1 teaspoon oil to fry pan. Turn fish over and brown other side for about 5 minutes. Cooking time depends on thickness of fish.

Sprinkle with lemon juice just before serving.

Fish Chowder

Makes 1 serving

> 1 teaspoon vegetable oil
> 2 tablespoons grated or chopped onion
> 1 medium potato, peeled and cut into small pieces
> ½ to 1 cup water
> ¾ cup milk
> 4 ounces (¼ lb) boneless cod, halibut, or other white fish, cut into small squares
> Salt and pepper to taste
> Thyme, if desired

Heat the oil in a medium size saucepan. Add onion and cook over low heat for about 2 minutes.

Add potato pieces and water. Cover tightly. Bring to a boil. Lower heat and simmer, until potatoes are cooked.

Add milk. Cook, stirring to prevent sticking, until milk is hot.

Add cut-up fish and seasonings. Cover and simmer over low heat 5 to 10 minutes or until fish is cooked.

Main Dish Lima Bean-Cheese Quickie

Makes 1 serving

> ⅔ cup of frozen lima beans
> ⅓ cup of tomato sauce
> 1 ounce (¼ cup) of American cheese, cut into small pieces

Cook lima beans in as little salted water as possible, drain, add tomato sauce. If you like "soupy" food, add a little extra sauce.

Cook over medium heat until hot. Stir in cut-up cheese and continue to cook only until cheese melts. Cover. Allow to stand a minute. Serve.

Chopped Liver Spread

for Salad Plate, Sandwich, or Snack

Makes 1 serving

>1 to 2 teaspoons of vegetable oil
>1 tablespoon of finely chopped onion
>1 raw chicken liver, cut into four or five pieces (use scissors to cut)
>½ teaspoon of mayonnaise
>Salt and pepper to taste

In a small fry pan, heat vegetable oil over medium heat. Add onion and cook for about 2 minutes or until tender but not browned.

Add liver pieces and cook until deep red changes color. Then mash liver with a fork.

Continue to cook, stirring as needed, until liver is done. Remove from heat. Allow to cool.

Add ½ teaspoon mayonnaise. Mix well. If necessary, add just a small amount of additional mayonnaise to make a smooth spread.

Spread on a slice of whole wheat bread and top with three or four raw spinach, escarole, or chicory leaves and remaining bread.

>**Note.** Because of the fat in the liver as well as the fat used to cook onion, it isn't necessary to coat bread with a spread.

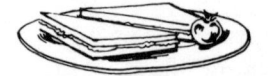

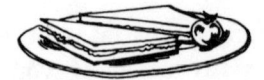

Cottage Cheese Combo Sandwiches

Cottage cheese combos may be used as a sandwich spread, as part of a salad plate, or a snack. Some of the more popular combos are:

Garden Combo. ¼ cup of cottage cheese combined and mixed with ¼ cup of chopped carrot, celery and/or green pepper.

Pickle Perker. ¼ cup of cottage cheese mixed with 1 tablespoon of chopped pickle.

Peanut Butter Combo. ¼ cup of cottage cheese combined and mixed with 2 level tablespoons of peanut butter.

Vegie Combo. ¼ cup of cottage cheese combined with ¼ cup of cooked mixed vegetables.

Tomato Teaser. ¼ cup of cottage cheese mixed with ¼ cup of chopped tomato.

White Sauce for Creamed Dishes

Makes about ½ cup

> 1½ teaspoons of fat
> 1 tablespoon of flour
> Sprinkling of salt and pepper
> ¼ cup of chicken or other pan drippings
> ¼ cup of milk

Melt fat in a small sauce or fry pan over medium heat. Stir in flour, salt and pepper to form smooth paste.

Add pan drippings and milk. Stir constantly while cooking. Cook until thickened.

Note. When you are cutting down on the use of fat, just mix well the flour, salt, drippings, and milk. Cook over medium to low heat until thickened.

Variations
1. Chicken, beef, or vegetable broth may be used in place of pan drippings
2. Add chopped parsley, if desired
3. Add dry mustard or curry powder
4. Add finely grated raw carrot

"From Scratch" Pizza

Note. Making two crusts at once gives you a second "From Scratch" Pizza for later that is as easy to prepare as the Nearly "no Work" Pizza.

Makes 2 9-inch pizzas

Dough

1½ cups of sifted enriched all-purpose flour, approximately
½ package (¼ ounce size) of active dry yeast
⅛ teaspoon of salt
½ cup of very warm (not hot) water
1 tablespoon vegetable oil

Measure into a medium size bowl ½ cup of flour, yeast and salt. Stir until thoroughly mixed.

Add water and vegetable oil. Beat by hand with hand beater for 2 minutes.

Stir in another ½ cup of flour. Beat until well mixed.

Continue to add 1 tablespoon at a time, stirring and turning after each addition, just enough additional flour to make a soft dough that pulls away from the sides of bowl.

On lightly floured hard surface knead dough until smooth and elastic, about 8 to 10 minutes.

Place dough in a bowl lightly greased with oil, turn dough over to grease other side. Cover the bowl with a clean dish towel. Let rise in a warm place, free from drafts, (do not place on radiator or stove) until double in size, about 45 minutes to 1 hour.

Prepare topping ingredients while dough is rising.

Topping for 1 9-inch pizza.

½ cup of tomato sauce
¼ teaspoon of crushed oregano leaves
Salt and pepper to taste
4 ounces of sliced and cubed mozzarella cheese
2 teaspoons of grated Parmesan cheese
2 teaspoons of oil

Combine in a small saucepan the sauce, oregano, salt and pepper. Heat until hot. Set aside.

Cut dough in half. Place halves of dough on lightly floured hard surface. Shape each into round ball. Flatten balls by slapping hard with the palms of hands. Using a rolling pin or your hands, shape flattened dough to fit the bottom of greased 9-inch pie pans. Place shaped dough in pans and gently stretch dough about ½ inch up the sides of pie pans.

Spoon and spread ½ the tomato sauce over one of the 9-inch pizza rounds. Top with the mozzarella cheese.

Spoon remaining sauce over mozzarella. Sprinkle with grated Parmesan cheese. Sprinkle with additional oregano to taste.

Drizzle with vegetable oil.

Place pizza as well as plain pizza round in a preheated 400° F. oven. Bake plain round for 15 minutes. Remove from oven.

Bake pizza about 15 minutes longer or until top is hot and bubbly and crust is golden brown and crisp-tender.

Place plain baked round on wire rack. Cool. May be refrigerated up to one week. To freeze, wrap in airtight material and freeze. To use, remove from refrigerator or freezer. Allow to reach room temperature. Spread with topping and cook at 400° F. Bake 25 minutes, or until done.

Nearly "No Work" Pizza

Makes 1 regular serving or 2 small servings

> 2 slices of whole wheat or enriched white bread toasted on one side (use broiler)
> ¼ to ⅓ cup of tomato sauce
> 2 ounces of mozzarella cheese, sliced and cut into small squares
> 2 teaspoons of grated Parmesan cheese
> 1 teaspoon of oil
> Oregano, to taste
> Salt, to taste

Place toasted side of bread on broiler rack or cookie sheet. Spread each slice of bread with about 1 tablespoon of tomato sauce. Sprinkle lightly with oregano. Top each slice with half the mozzarella cheese. Spoon about 1 tablespoon of tomato sauce over mozzarella on each slice bread. Sprinkle with Parmesan cheese and salt. Drizzle oil over each slice. Sprinkle lightly with oregano.

Place under broiler and broil only until topping is hot and bubbly and cheese is very soft. Watch carefully to avoid burning.

Variation. Use hard roll or English muffins split in two instead of bread. No need to toast.

Note. If you would rather not use broiler, the Nearly "No Work" Pizza may be baked in a hot oven until topping is hot and bubbly, and cheese is very soft.

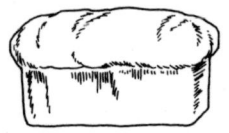

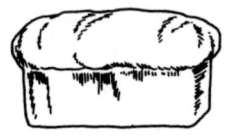

No-Knead White Bread

Makes 1 loaf

>¾ cup of warm (not hot) water
>1 package of active dry yeast
>2 tablespoons of honey, sugar, or molasses
>1 teaspoon of salt
>2 tablespoons of vegetable oil
>¾ cup warm (not hot) milk
>3½ cups of sifted enriched all-purpose flour
>
>**Note.** Warm water is 105° F. to 115° F.

Measure into a warm large mixing bowl the warm (not hot) water. (Never use hot water because it kills the yeast, which makes the bread rise.) Sprinkle in the yeast. Stir until dissolved. Stir in honey, salt, and vegetable oil. Add warm (not hot) milk and mix until well blended.

Add 1½ cups of flour. Beat 2 minutes at medium speed with electric beater or hand beater, or beat by hand for 3 to 4 minutes.

Stir in, by hand, only enough of the remaining flour to make a stiff dough.

If it is too difficult to stir in flour, you may want to use your hands to thoroughly mix the dough, which will be stiff and sticky.

Cover with a clean dish towel. Let rise in warm place, free from drafts, until doubled in size, about 50 minutes.

Using a spoon, stir batter down and beat for another ½ minute. Spread evenly in greased 9 x 5 x 3-inch loaf pan or greased 1½ quart casserole.

Cover with towel. Let rise in warm place, free from drafts, until double in size, about 30 minutes. (Do not allow to rise too much since this causes the bread to fall.)

Bake in a preheated oven at 375° F. for 45 to 50 minutes or until done. Remove from pan and cool on wire rack.

No-Knead Whole Wheat Bread

Makes 1 loaf

¾ cup of warm (not hot) water
1 package of active dry yeast
2 tablespoons of honey, sugar, or molasses
1 teaspoon of salt
2 tablespoons of vegetable oil
¾ cup of warm (not hot) milk
2 cups of unsifted whole wheat flour
1½ cups of sifted enriched all-purpose flour

Measure into a warm large mixing bowl the warm water. Never use *hot* water because it kills the yeast, which makes the bread rise. Sprinkle in the yeast. Stir until dissolved. Stir in honey, salt, and vegetable oil. Add warm (not hot) milk and mix until well blended.

Add 1½ cups of whole wheat flour. Beat 2 minutes at medium speed with an electric or hand beater, or beat by hand for 3 to 4 minutes.

Using a spoon, stir in remaining ½ cup of whole wheat flour and mix for about ½ minute. Stir in, by hand, only enough white flour to make a stiff dough.

If it is too difficult to stir in flour, you may want to use your hands to thoroughly mix the dough, which will be stiff and sticky.

Cover with a clean dish towel. Let rise in warm place, free from drafts, until doubled in size, about 50 minutes. Do not place on radiator or stove to rise.

Using a spoon, stir batter down. Spread evenly in greased 9 x 5 x 3-inch loaf pan or greased 1½ quart casserole.

Cover with towel. Let rise in warm place, free from drafts, until double in size, about 30 minutes. (Do not allow to rise too much since this causes the bread to fall.)

Bake in a preheated oven at 375° F. for 45 to 50 minutes or until done. Remove from pan and cool on wire rack.

Banana Bread

Makes 1 loaf (12 to 16 slices)

    1¾ cups of sifted enriched flour
    2 teaspoons of baking powder
    ¼ teaspoon of baking soda
    ½ teaspoon of salt
    ¼ cup of vegetable oil
    2 eggs, well beaten
    ½ cup of sugar
    1 teaspoon of vanilla
    ¾ teaspoon of lemon rind, if desired
    1 cup of well-mashed, very ripe banana

Preheat oven to 350 ° F.

Sift into a large bowl the flour, baking powder, baking soda, and salt.

In another bowl, combine and beat until well mixed and blended the oil, eggs, sugar, vanilla, and lemon rind. Stir in mashed banana. Add to flour mixture, stirring only until flour is moistened.

Spoon or pour into well-greased and lightly floured loaf pan. Spread evenly in pan.

Bake at 350° F. in preheated oven for 50 to 60 minutes. Bread is done when a toothpick inserted into the middle of bread comes out clean.

Cool in pan on wire rack for 10 minutes. Remove from pan. Place on wire rack and cool completely.

    Variation. Add ½ cup chopped nuts when bananas are added.

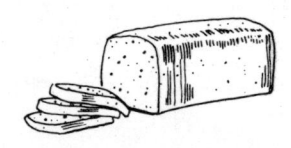

Top-of-Stove Bread Pudding

Makes 2 to 3 servings

> 2 slices of bread
> Margarine or butter, softened
> ⅔ cup of skim milk or regular whole milk
> 1 egg
> 2 tablespoons of sugar or brown sugar
> Vanilla extract, to taste
> Cinnamon or nutmeg, to taste
> Grated lemon rind, if desired

Lightly spread bread (white or whole wheat or raisin or cinnamon) with softened butter or margarine. Cut into small squares. Put bread in lightly greased top part of double boiler.

Measure milk into a large measuring cup. Add egg, sugar, and vanilla, cinnamon or nutmeg, and lemon rind. Beat until well blended. Pour over bread. Do not stir. Sprinkle lightly with additional spice. Cover.

Pour just enough hot water into the bottom of double boiler so that when water comes to a boil it does not touch pot holding the pudding. Bring water to a boil, and cook pudding over water until it is "set," about 30 minutes. A silver knife put into the center of the pudding should come out clean.

Turn off heat and allow pudding to stand 10 minutes before serving. May be served hot or cold.

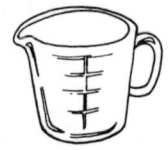

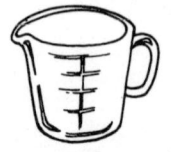

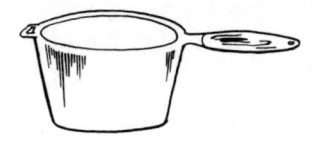

Brown Sugar Top-of-Stove Bread Pudding

Makes 2 to 3 servings

> 2 slices of bread
> Margarine or butter, softened
> 1½ to 2 tablespoons of firmly packed brown sugar
> ⅔ cup of milk
> 1 egg
> Vanilla extract, to taste
> Cinnamon or nutmeg, to taste

Lightly spread bread with margarine or butter. Cut into small cubes. Set aside. Spread brown sugar evenly over bottom of lightly-greased top pan of double boiler. Spoon or place bread cubes over sugar. Do not mix or stir.

Measure milk into a large measuring cup. Add egg, vanilla, and spice. Mix until well blended. Pour over bread. Do not stir or mix. Lightly sprinkle top with additional spice. Cover.

Pour just enough hot water into the bottom of double boiler so that when water comes to a boil it does not touch pot holding the pudding. Bring water to a boil, and cook pudding over water until it is "set," about 30 minutes. A silver knife put into the center of the pudding should come out clean.

Turn off heat and allow pudding to stand 10 minutes before serving. May be served hot or cold.

Pudding with Topping

Make your favorite homemade or packaged mix pudding, such as vanilla. If one package makes too much, measure out half the mix and use half the liquid to make a smaller amount.

When ready to use pudding, measure out ¼ to ½ cup of pudding into dessert dish or cup. Top with one of the following:

- 2 tablespoons of crumbled oatmeal cookies
- ½ peach or peach slices, cut into small pieces with a sprinkling of chopped nuts
- 2 tablespoons of drained crushed pineapple and a sprinkling of cookie crumbs
- 2 to 3 tablespoons of crumbled banana or nut bread

No-Cook Prunes

1 cup of dried prunes
2 cups of water

Place prunes and water in a container. Cover. Place in refrigerator for three to four days. After two days check and add more water if necessary. As the prunes stand the water becomes dark and sweet. If you want a thick sauce allow to stand longer than five days.

Use the prunes and juice as a breakfast fruit, as dessert, in salads, and snack food.

Variations
1. Add cinnamon to taste
2. Add lemon juice to taste
3. Add 1 tablespoon of honey
4. Instead of dried prunes use ¼ cup of raisins, ½ cup of prunes, and ¼ cup of apricots

Recommended Reading

THE FOLLOWING PUBLICATIONS are available from the United States Government Printing Office, Superintendent of Documents, Washington, D.C. 20402. Prices shown were in effect at the time this book was being written. Government documents' prices are subject to change without prior notice. Therefore, prices in effect when your order is filled may differ from the prices below. Order by the numbers listed and title of publication.

Nutrition

Conserving the Nutritive Value in Foods. Rev. 1971 (16 pp.).

    A 1.77:90/3   001-000-00869-2   35¢

Fats in Food and Diet. 1976 (12 pp.).

    A 1.75:361/3   001-000-03568-1   35¢

Key Nutrients. Rev. 1971 (4 pp.).

    A 1.68:691/2   001-000-01492-7   35¢

Nutrition Labeling, Tools for its Use. Contains information that supplements what is on food labels. You get a table showing amounts of calories, proteins, vitamins, and minerals supplied by 900 foods; a table showing the amounts of nutrients recommended for men, women, and children of different ages; and lists of foods that are important sources of specific nutrients. 1975 (57 pp.).

    A 1.75:382   001-000-03385-9 $1.15

Nutritive Value of American Foods in Common Units. Tells you how many calories and nutrients are in common units of each of approximately 1500 foods. The nutrients measured are water, food, energy, protein, fat, carbohydrates, five mineral elements (iron, calcium, phosphorus, sodium, potassium), five vitamins (including vitamin A), total saturated fatty acids, and two unsaturated fatty acids. Three appendixes contain additional data on the composition of foods and on weight-volume relationships among foods. 1975 (291 pp.).

    A 1.76:456   001-000-03184-8 $5.15

Nutritive Value of Foods. Rev. 1977 (40 pp.).

    A 1.77:72/5   001-000-03-667-0 $1.05

Raw, Processed, Prepared. Includes information useful in estimating the nutrient values of food and presents 5 tables of data on composition of foods—edible portions of 100 grams, edible portions of 1 pound as purchased, selected fatty acids, cholesterol and magnesium content. Data is given for energy, proximate composition, vitamin A, thiamine, riboflavin, niacin, ascorbic acid, calcium, phosphorus, iron, sodium, and potassium. 1963, reprinted 1976 (190 pp.).

    A 1.76:8/963   001-000-00768-8 $3.60

Purchasing, Storing, and Preparing Foods

Freezing Combination Main Dishes. This booklet outlines the types of food, equipment, and packaging materials required to freeze your meals. It includes 16 pages of tempting recipes for such freezable main dishes as American lasagna, chicken a la king, ham turnovers, and turkey-macaroni casserole. Rev. 1976 (22 pp.).

    A 1.77:40/5   001-000-03559-2   40¢

Freezing Meat and Fish in the Home. Provides information on general freezing, wrapping, storage, and thawing procedures, cutting methods, boning the cuts of meat, fish selection, cleaning, dressing, and more. Rev. 1973 (23 pp.).

    A 1.77:93/7   001-000-02981-9   55¢

Home Canning of Fruits and Vegetables. Describes the various types of canning equipment that can be used, and provides illustrated instructions for canning of more than 30 different fruits and vegetables. Rev. 1976 (32 pp.).

    A 1.77:8/10   001-000-03535-5   45¢

Home Canning of Meat and Poultry. Provides easy-to-follow directions for the canning of poultry, rabbit, beef, veal, pork, lamb, and other meats. 1972 (24 pp.).

    A 1.77:106/5   001-000-02612-7   35¢

Home Care of Purchased Frozen Foods. Provides advice on temperature, length of storage, and types of food best suited for frozen storage. Includes a chart of maximum home storage periods for purchased frozen food. 1975 (6 pp.).

    A 1.77:69/6   001-000-03410-3   35¢

Home Freezing of Fruits and Vegetables. Includes illustrated directions for freezing many fruits and vegetables so they retain their freshness and nutritive value. Also tells what fruits and vegetables can be frozen, how to prepare them, what type of containers to use, and how to use them properly. 1971, reprinted 1976 (48 pp.).

    A 1.77:10/7   001-000-02448-5   75¢

FEEL BETTER AFTER 50 FOOD BOOK • 210

Home Freezing of Poultry and Poultry Main Dishes. Contains directions for freezing raw and cooked poultry, as well as recipes for combination poultry main dishes and salads suitable for freezing. Rev. 1975 (29 pp.).

    A 1.75:371   001-000-03284-4   50¢

It's Good Food—Keep It Safe. 1973 (6 pp.).

    A 1.68:1057   001-000-02953-3   35¢

Keeping Foods Clean. 1974 (4 pp.).

    HE 20.4010/A:F 739/3   017-012-00217-0   35¢

Keeping Food Safe to Eat: A Guide for Homemakers. 1975 (11 pp.).

    A 1.77:162/3   001-000-03396-4   35¢

Storing Perishable Foods in the Home. Gives specific directions on how to handle, prepare for storage, and store a wide variety of foods. Includes information on caring for perishable foods in the home so that nutritive value, quality, and flavor are preserved. Rev. 1973 (12 pp.).

    A 1.77:78/5   001-000-02715-8   35¢

Storing Vegetables and Fruits in Basements, Cellars, Outbuildings, and Pits. Tips on how to do it right. Rev. 1973 (18 pp.).

    A 1.77:119/3   001-000-02942-8   40¢

Vegetables in Family Meals, A Guide For Customers. Contains practical tips on buying and storing vegetables, cooking vegetables, enhancing their flavor, and using leftovers. Rev. 1975 (36 pp.).

    A 1.77:105/6   001-000-03271-2   45¢

What to do When Your Home Freezer Stops. 1972, reprinted 1975 (8 pp.)

    A 1.35:321/4   001-000-02840-5   35¢

Index

Aging and nutrition, 7, 103
Amino acids, 41–42, 70, 72
Amounts of servings, 36–37
  of breads and cereals, 81
  of meat and meat alternates, 79
  of milk foods, 81
  of vegetables and fruits, 80
Anemia and nutritional deficiencies, 62, 63, 72, 75
Appetite loss and thiamine deficiency, 66
Apples (*see also* Fruits)
  buying and storage of, 135, 136
Apricots (*see also* Fruits)
  buying and storage of, 135, 136
Asparagus (*see also* Vegetables)
  as raw food, 11, 133
Atherosclerosis, 50–51
Avocados
  calories in, 113
  storage time, 136

Banana bread (recipe), 203
Bananas (*see also* Fruits)
  breakfast drink with, 29–30
  buying and storage of, 134–135
  overripe, use of, 135
Beans, dry (*see also* Legumes)
  chili con carne, 27, 45
  nutrients in, 46, 75
Beans, green (*see* Vegetables)
Beans, lima, with cheese (recipe), 195
Bedtime snacks, 28

Beef (*see also* Meats)
  broth, preparation of, 153
  buying tips, 95, 149–151
  chuck steak, money-saving use of, 149–154
  ground, *see* Hamburger
  nutrients in, 45, 75–76
Blood building nutrients, 42, 43, 63, 72, 73
Blood clotting
  and calcium, 10, 73
  and vitamin C, 12
  and vitamin K, 61
Blood lipids (fats), 50
Blood sugar and energy, 53
Body fat, role of, 49
Body functioning and nutrients
  carbohydrates, 52–55
  fats, 48–49
  minerals, 73–77
  protein, 40–43
  vitamin A, 58–59
  vitamin B complex, 64–73
  vitamin C, 63
  vitamin D, 60–61
  vitamin K, 61
  water, 56–57
Body temperature and water, 57
Bones, nutrients for, 40, 42, 58, 61, 63, 77
Brain, nutrients for, 40, 42
Bran, 56, 128
Bread and rolls
  calories in, 9, 114
  as fiber source, 55
  as starch source, 53

storage of, 145
vitamins and minerals in, 9, 65, 67, 69, 70, 71, 76
whole grain, 9–10, 14, 32, 55
Bread making (recipes), 201–203
Bread pudding, top-of-stove (recipe), 204–205
Breakfast, 26–30
  feel-better drink for (recipe), 30
Breathing difficulty and thiamine deficiency, 66
Broccoli (*see also* Vegetables)
  as convenience food, 183
  preparation of, 143–144
  as raw food, 11, 133
  in salad, 90, 143
  vitamins and minerals in, 11, 143
Butter (*see also* Milk foods)
  nutrients in, 51, 60

Cabbage (*see also* Vegetables)
  buying and storage of, 138
  coleslaw, 12
  vitamins in, 62, 64, 80, 138
Calcium, 10, 73–74
  foods that affect use of, 74, 78
  sources of, 10, 11, 16, 29, 44, 73–74
  supplement for vegetarians, 72
  USRDA adjusted for aging, 180
Calories
  daily allowances of, 105, 180
  empty, in sweets, 15–16, 23, 54, 110
  in fried foods, 15
  intake of, and age, 7
  intake of, and weight gain, 123
  listing of, by individual foods, 110–123
  and protein, 42, 43
Canned foods, buying and storage of, 166–169
Carbohydrates, 40, 52–55
  and B vitamins, 65, 70, 72
  and calories, 43, 52
  and fiber, *see* Fiber
  forms of, 52–53
Carotene, 59, 78
Carrots (*see also* Vegetables)
  as fiber source, 55
  sticks, preparation of, 131–132
  as vitamin A source, 59
Cauliflower (*see also* Vegetables)
  raw, preparation of, 133
Cereals
  as bedtime snack, 28
  calories in, 9, 114–115
  as fiber source, 9–10, 54, 56, 128
  nutrients in, 9, 41, 46, 53, 65, 66, 68, 70, 71
  package labels on, 177–178
  ready-sweetened, 177–178
  serving suggestions, 88
  shopping for, 185–186
Cheese (*see also* Milk foods)
  calories in, 110
  cream, 20
  and macaroni, baked, 28, 44, 193
  nutrients in, 10, 16, 20, 41, 44, 60, 84–85
  sliced, cost of, 183
  storage of, 147–148
  in vegetarian diets, 44
Cheese-lima bean main dish (recipe), 195
Chewing problems, 160–161
Chicken (*see also* Poultry)

ground, for loaf or meatballs, 161
money-saving cutting plan for, 154–159
prepared coatings for, 182–183
recipes for, 190–191
as source of nutrients, 41, 45, 51, 69, 71
Chocolate, hidden fat in, 48
Cholesterol, 49–51
Citrus fruits (*see also* Fruits)
buying tips on, 137
calories in, 113
frozen juice concentrate, 136–137, 184
season for, 187
storage of, 137
as vitamin C source, 64, 80, 136–137
Coffee, 28, 51–52
Cold cuts, 18, 184–185
Constipation and diet, 124–129
laxatives, 129
Convenience foods, cost of, 181–185
Cottage cheese (*see also* Milk foods)
as protein source, 46, 84
sandwiches, recipes for, 196–197
Cream, 49, 51
substitutes for, 51–52
Creamed foods
contamination hazards of, 163
sauce for (recipe), 197
Cutting board, food contamination from, 164

Daily Food Guide, U.S. Dept. of Agriculture, 79–85
Depression and B vitamins, 65
Diabetes and diet, 25, 102
Diarrhea and diet, 43
Diets, restricted, 25, 107, 108, 166
Disease, resistance to, and nutrients, 42–43, 58
Diverticulitis and raw foods, 11–12
Dry mouth and vitamin A, 58

Egg-fry and spinach dish (recipe), 194
Eggs
for breakfast, 28–30
fats in, 48
as source of nutrients, 41, 44, 48, 59, 60, 61, 71, 72, 76, 79
in vegetarian diets, 44
Elimination (*see also* Constipation; Diarrhea)
and fiber, 8, 10, 55
and raw foods, 11–12
and water, 87
Enemas, abuse of, 125
Energy and nutrients, 7, 12–14, 42, 43, 49, 52–53, 57
Enzymes, role in body, 42
Exercise, benefits of, 109, 125, 127
Eyesight and vitamin A, 58

Fast foods as nourishment, 13–16
Fat cells and body weight, 103
Fats, 40, 46–52
and elimination problems, 128–129
"hidden" sources of, 48, 82
interaction with vitamins, 49, 58, 62, 70, 72
in reducing diets, 106
saturated and unsaturated, 47–48, 50, 51
as source of calories, 43, 48, 111

Fiber, 54, 55, 56
  sources of, 8, 10, 54–56, 83, 128
Fish and shellfish
  calories in, 112
  canned, 167
  frozen, handling of, 165
  nutrients in, 41, 45, 46, 48, 61, 68, 69, 71, 72, 77
  storage time of, 165
Fish, pan-fried (recipe), 194
Fish chowder (recipe), 195
Food Finder, 39–78
Food grinders, use of, 160–161
  as source of contamination, 164
Food poisoning, 161–166
Frankfurters, 22, 112
Fried foods, 15, 51, 58
Frozen foods
  cheese, 147–148
  fruit juices, 136–137
  meats and fish, 153–154, 165
  vegetables, 140–141
Fruits
  buying tips on, 133–138, 187–188
  calories in, 113–114
  drinks, ingredients in, 178, 184
  fiber content of, 11, 55–56, 128
  juices, 136–137, 184
  for reducing diets, 106
  storage of, 134–138, 209–210
  vitamins in, 59–60, 62, 64–65, 71, 80
Fruits, dried, 54, 128
  calories in, 114
  nutrients in, 71, 76

Gelatine, protein in, 41
Grains, *see* Cereals
Gravies, contamination hazards of, 163

Hair, nutrients for, 42, 59
Ham (*see also* Meat, Pork)
  nutrients in, 45, 66
Hamburger as source of nourishment, 13–15, 18, 22–23
Heart action, nutrients to promote, 65, 73
Heart disease and diet, 50–51
  (*see also* Hypertension)
Hormones, production of, 42, 50
Hypertension, 102, 108

Infections, resistance to, and nutrition, 8, 42–43, 63
Iodine, sources of, 77
Iron, 42, 74–75
  sources of, 9, 11, 21, 44, 73, 75–76, 83
  supplement for vegetarians, 72
  USRDA adjusted for aging, 180
  and vitamin C, 63, 78
Irritability and B vitamin deficiencies, 65, 72

Jams and jellies, 53
Joint pains
  and vitamin A, 59
  and vitamin C, 12

Kale (*see also* Vegetables)
  buying and use of, 139
Knives, care of, 154
  food contamination from, 164

Labels on food packages, reading of, 10, 18, 22, 81, 83, 177–180
Lard, 47
Laxatives, 125, 129
Leftovers, use of, 27, 93

Legumes
  calories in, 117
  as fiber source, 128
  nutrients in, 41, 53, 66, 67,
    68, 70, 71, 73, 75, 77, 79
Lentils (*see* Legumes)
Life expectancy and weight,
  102
Lima bean-cheese main dish
  (recipe), 195
Liver (*see also* Meat)
  chopped spread (recipe), 196
  nutrients in, 45, 59, 61, 66–
    69, 72, 73, 75, 83
Liver trouble and nutrition, 43
Lunch, 20–25

Macaroni
  calories in, 115
  nutrients in, 53, 67, 68, 85
  in vegetarian diets, 44
Macaroni and cheese (top-of-
    stove recipe), 193
  for breakfast, 28
  calories in, 115
  as protein source, 84–85
Magnesium, 77
Margarine, 47–49, 60, 62, 81
Mayonnaise, 48
Meat
  buying and use, money-
    saving plan for, 149–154
  calories in, 112
  cold cuts, 18, 184–185
  frozen, 165
  nutrients in, 41, 44–46, 66–
    69, 71, 72, 75–76, 83
  prepared, cost of, 184, 192
  storage time for, 164–165
Meat by-products, 22
Meat loaf (recipe), 192
Melons
  storage time, 136
  vitamins in, 59, 60, 64, 80

Men
  calorie allowance for, 105
  weight of, 102, 104
Menu suggestions, 14, 19, 21,
    24
  for five-a-day meals, 37–38
  for reducing diets, 107
  for three-a-day meals, 32–33,
    88–101
Milk foods
  allergies to, 10
  breakfast drink with, 28
  calories in, 9, 16, 110–111
  forms of, 146–147
  nutrients in, 10, 16, 41, 44,
    60, 67–70, 72–74, 78, 83
Milk pudding with topping
    (recipe), 206
Mineral oil, 52, 129
Minerals, 40, 73–77
  sources of, 73–77, 83
Mucus membrane and
    vitamin A, 58
Muscle functioning and
    nutrients, 10, 42, 43, 65,
    73–75

Nails, condition of, and protein,
    42
Nausea and thiamine
    deficiency, 66
Nerves, health of, nutrients for,
    10, 40, 42, 65, 69
Niacin, 69–70
  sources of, 9, 11, 69–70, 83
  USRDA adjusted for aging,
    180
Night blindness and vitamin A,
    48
Nitrites in food, 22
Noodles
  calories in, 116
  nutrients in, 46, 53, 67, 68

Numbness and thiamine
  deficiency, 66
Nutrition labeling, 10, 179–180
Nuts
  calories in, 117
  nutrients in, 41, 62, 68, 71,
    77, 79

Oils, vegetable, 47–49
  and mineral oil, 52
  as vitamin E source, 62
Oranges (*see* Citrus fruits)

Packaged mixes, 82, 182–183
Packaging
  Labels, *see* Labels on food
    packages
  traps, 181, 185–189
Peaches (*see also* Fruits)
  buying and storage of, 135,
    136
  calories in, 113
  cooking of, 135
  season for, 187, 188
Peanut Butter (*see also*
    Peanuts)
  calories in, 117
  as fattening food, 123
  "hidden" fat in, 48
Peanut butter-cottage cheese
    combo (recipe), 197
Peanuts
  calories in, 117
  nutrients in, 46, 62, 70, 71, 73
Pears (*see* Fruits)
Peas, dried (*see also* Legumes)
  calories in, 117
  soup, canned, 20, 21, 74
Peas, green (*see also*
    Vegetables)
  as raw food, 11
  in salads, 11
  soup, canned, 20, 21
Peppers (*see also* Vegetables)

  buying tips, 132–133
  ready-to-eat sticks, 132–133
Phosphorus, 77
  and calcium absorption, 78
Pickle-cottage cheese combo
    (recipe), 197
Pizza
  commercial and homemade,
    16–18
  recipes for, 198–200
Pork (*see also* Ham; Meat)
  canned, 168
  nutrients in, 45, 65, 66, 73, 76
  sausage, 48
Potato chips, 120, 123
Potatoes
  buying and storage of, 138–
    139
  calories in, 120
  cooking methods, 15, 89
  as fiber source, 55, 56
  nutrients in, 12, 53, 59, 64,
    71, 80, 138
Potatoes, sweet
  calories in, 121
  nutrients in, 53, 59, 71
Poultry (*see also* Chicken)
  calories in, 112
  frozen, handling of, 165
  nutrients in, 68, 69, 71
  stuffings for, spoilage
    problems of, 163
Preparation of food (*see also*
    Recipes)
  beef broth, 53
  cooked fruits, 135
  cooked vegetables, 140, 144
  fix-ahead raw vegetables,
    131–133
  preservation of vitamins in,
    60, 63–64
Preservatives in food, 22
Protein, 41–46
  amount needed, 44–45, 180

complete and incomplete, 21, 41–42
foods rich in, 44–46
in vegetarian diets, 44
Prunes (*see also* Fruits), 32, 36
no-cook (recipe), 206
Pudding with topping (recipe), 206

Reading materials, 207–211
Recipes
banana bread, 203
bread pudding, 204–205
breads, 201–202
breakfast drink, 30–31
chicken dishes, 190–191
chopped liver spread, 196
cottage cheese combo sandwiches, 196–197
fish dishes, 194–195
lima bean-cheese main dish, 195
macaroni and cheese top-of-stove main dish, 193
meat loaf and meat balls, 192
pizzas, 198–200
prunes, no-cook, 206
puddings, 204–205, 206
sauce for creamed foods, 197
spinach and egg-fry dish, 194
Reducing diet, menus for (table), 107
Riboflavin, 68–69
sources of, 9, 10, 11, 16, 68–69, 83
USRDA adjusted for aging, 180
Rice
calories in, 116
and chicken, 88, 190
as fiber source, 56
nutrients in, 46, 53
Roughage (*see* Fiber)

Salad dressing, 49, 163

Salads, 11, 27, 90, 141–143
Salt
foods high in, 18, 22, 108
restricted diets, 25, 108, 166
Sandwiches, 20–21, 27
cottage cheese fillings for (recipe), 196–197
Sardines, canned, 167
Sauce
commercial mixes for, 182
for creamed dishes, 197
spoilage problems of, 163
Shopping for food, 170–189
for canned foods, 168–169
for fruit, 133–135, 137–138
and label reading, *see* Labels on food packages
for vegetables, 138–141
Sinus trouble, 58
Skin health and nutrients, 42, 49, 59, 68, 69
Soft drinks, 15–16, 23, 54, 110, 122
Soybeans (*see also* Legumes)
nutrients in, 46, 62
Spaghetti, nutrients in, 22, 45, 46, 53, 67, 68
Spinach (*see also* Vegetables)
and egg fry (recipe), 194
as iron source, 75
storage and cooking, 139–140
Staples, checklist of, 172
Starch (*see* Carbohydrates)
Storage of food, 132–148, 161–169
for preservation of vitamins, 60, 63–64
Strawberries (*see also* Fruits)
buying tips, 138
storage of, 136, 138
Sugar (*see also* Carbohydrates), 9, 52, 53, 82, 123

Supplementation of nutrients, 44, 54
Sweets, empty calories in, 23, 54, 123
Swelling and nutritional deficiencies, 43, 59

Teeth and gums, health of, and nutrition, 11, 40, 58, 61, 63, 73, 77
Thiamine, 65–68
  sources of, 11, 66–68, 83
  USRDA adjusted for aging, 180
Tomato-cottage cheese combo, 197
Triglycerides and heart disease, 50
Tuna, canned, 20–21, 45, 167
TV dinners, 82

Unit pricing, 181, 185–186
USRDA standards for nutrients, 10, 45–46, 59–60, 64, 66–70, 73–76, 179–181

Vegetable-cottage cheese combo (recipe), 197
Vegetables
  buying and storage of, 138–145
  cooking of, 140, 144–145
  as fiber source, 8, 11, 54–56
  leafy, 8, 139–143
  as mineral source, 74–76
  oils from, 47–49, 62
  as protein source, 41
  raw, 11–12, 131–133
  salads, 11, 27, 90, 141–143
  as vitamin source, 8, 59–62, 64, 65, 67, 68, 70, 71, 73, 80
Vegetarian diets, 44, 72
Vitamin A, 8, 58–60, 180
  fat-solubility, 49, 52, 58, 60
  sources of, 8, 11, 59, 64–65, 80, 83, 132, 141–142
  and vitamin E, 78
Vitamin B complex (*see also* Niacin; Riboflavin; Thiamine)
  B_6, 70, 71
  B_{12}, 44, 71–72
  USRDA adjusted for aging, 180
Vitamin C, 12, 63–64, 180
  and iron, 63, 78
  sources of, 11–12, 64–65, 80, 83, 136–318
Vitamin D, 60–61
  and calcium, 61, 78
  fat solubility, 49, 52, 58, 60
Vitamin E, 62
  fat solubility, 49, 52, 58
  and vitamin A, 78
Vitamin K, 61–62
  fat solubility, 49, 52, 58

Water, need of body for, 40, 56–57, 127
  sodium in, 166
Water balance of body, 10, 43
Water retention, 57
Weight, normal and abnormal, 102–104
Weight loss and vitamin deficiency, 59, 63
Weight watching, 102–123
  and calories, *see* Calories
  and carbohydrates, 52, 55
  and exercise, 109
  menus for, 107
Wheat germ, 56, 62
Women
  calorie allowance for, 105
  weight of, 102, 104

Zinc for vegetarians, 44, 72
Zucchini as raw food, 11, 133